THE
HEALTH PROFESSIONAL'S GUIDE
TO
WRITING FOR PUBLICATION

THE
HEALTH PROFESSIONAL'S GUIDE
TO
WRITING FOR PUBLICATION

By

RHODA WEISS-LAMBROU

Associate Professor of Occupational Therapy
Ecole de réadaptation
"School of Rehabilitation"
Université de Montréal

With a Foreword by

Geraldine Moore, O.T. (C).

Editor of the Canadian Journal of Occupational Therapy

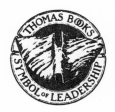

C H A R L E S   C   T H O M A S   •   P U B L I S H E R
Springfield • Illinois • U.S.A.

Published and Distributed Throughout the World by

CHARLES C THOMAS • PUBLISHER
2600 South First Street
Springfield, Illinois 62794-9265

© *1989 by* CHARLES C THOMAS • PUBLISHER

ISBN 0-398-05592-0

Library of Congress Catalog Card Number: 89-4396

With THOMAS BOOKS *careful attention is given to all details of manufacturing
and design. It is the Publisher's desire to present books that are satisfactory as to their
physical qualities and artistic possibilities and appropriate for their particular use.
THOMAS BOOKS will be true to those laws of quality that assure a good name
and good will.*

Printed in the United States of America
SC-R-3

Library of Congress Cataloging-in-Publication Data

Weiss-Lambrou, Rhoda.
    The health professional's guide to writing for publication / Rhoda
Weiss-Lambrou ; with a foreword by Geraldine Moore.
       p. cm.
    Includes bibliographies and index.
    ISBN 0-398-05592-0
    1. Medical writing.   I. Title.
    [DNLM: 1. Publishing.   2. Writing.   WZ 345 W433h]
RT119.W45   1989
808'.06661—dc 19
DNLM/DLC
For Library of Congress   89-4396
                                            CIP

To my mother and father

FOREWORD

Today the communication process has assumed an important and sophisticated role in our society. The ability to communicate our thoughts and ideas, and to share our knowledge with others, is also of paramount importance. It is one of the yardsticks by which we are measured. From an early age, verbal communication skills are emphasized and other communication skills are assimulated in quick succession, with varying degrees of success.

It is a well accepted fact that knowledge gained by research and in practice more than doubles its value when shared with others who can put it to use. As health care practitioners, whether involved in research, education, administration or clinical practice, the knowledge we gain from our experience or the findings of our research are invaluable pieces of information for our colleagues. It is only by sharing and communicating this knowledge that it can be authenticated and be considered a valued contribution.

Since Gutenberg and Caxton in the mid-fifteenth century, communicating knowledge in the written and printed form has always been considered the accepted and most permanent form of record. Although today the computer screen is a well accepted adjunct, this knowledge still has to be disseminated in an intelligent, coherent, and organized manner for its true value to be realized.

In many scientific fields, the ability to publish successfully is considered the final completion of education. *The Health Professional's Guide to Writing for Publication* is an important and valuable part of this education process. It is written for those who wish to contribute to the body of knowledge of their profession. It is written for those who have a wealth of experience and expertise to share with colleagues. It guides the fledgling author through the myriad of do's and don't's of writing, as well as the maze of various instructions published by editors of journals, like myself. It counsels and informs those who already have some experience with the publication process. Another person's insights and experience easily translates to good advice.

vii

Most of all, *The Health Professional's Guide to Writing for Publication* motivates. It tells you where to start; it also tells you when to stop. Whether you pick up your pen, or place your fingers on the keyboard, this book encourages and motivates you to get on with the task of writing. I am really looking forward to reaping the benefits of all the hard work done by Rhoda Weiss-Lambrou. This major contribution to publishing for the health professions will be appreciated by editors waiting to receive those well written manuscripts, equally as much as those who read the book. Take her advice, and write.

Geraldine Moore, O.T.(C).
Editor of the *Canadian Journal of Occupational Therapy*

PREFACE

Do you wish to contribute to the scientific and clinical body of knowledge in the field of health science by writing a journal or book publication?

Have you considered becoming involved in the scientific writing process but did not feel that you knew how to prepare and write a manuscript for journal publication?

Do you have an idea and material for writing a book but do not know how to find and approach a publisher?

Have you submitted a manuscript for publication to a journal only to have it rejected?

If you are a health professional who has answered yes to any of these questions, reading this book will be your guide to writing better manuscripts and to achieving the goal of publication. The primary purpose of the book is to help health professionals write a journal or book-length manuscript that has a greater potential for being published. This audience of health practitioners includes primarily occupational and physical therapists, as well as speech therapists, social workers, psychologists, nurses and doctors. Undergraduate and graduate students in any of the health care professions may also find this book useful when preparing a manuscript for publication.

In the health science literature, a large number of journal publications and books are written by health professionals who are prominent researchers and academics. In general, these authors acquired much of their scientific writing skills in the course of their graduate work, and today often produce scholarly publications in order to contend with the "publish or perish" phenomenon inherent in the university system. Although most researchers and academics have the writing skills required to getting published, there are times however that the pressure to publish may result in their preparing papers which do not meet the criteria for publication.

Unlike academics and researchers, clinicians comprise the majority of the health professional workforce and are not obliged by their work setting to write for publication. As a result, there are those health practitioners who are not interested in becoming an author and there are those who aspire to writing a journal article or book but do not know how to write one that is of a publishable nature. There are of course clinicians who are able to write quality papers that are published; however, I feel that a greater number of health practitioners should and could write for publication, if they learned to develop their writing and publishing potential.

Health professionals have an important contribution to make to the scientific and clinical body of knowledge in their field. From their clinical experiences, many clinicians have developed new ideas and approaches that would be of value and interest to their colleagues. A publication in the form of a journal article or book is a means of sharing this knowledge and of expanding one's competencies. Unlike a conference presentation at a professional or scientific meeting, a publication serves as a more permanent document for describing existing practices, reviewing past knowledge or providing empirical research.

For several years, I have been on the review board of the *Canadian Journal of Occupational Therapy* and have acted as a consulting reviewer for three health professional journals. I believe that although health practitioners are well-prepared for their professional practice, many do not have the writing skills required for producing publishable manuscripts. They have difficulty preparing coherent and well-organized papers, and as a result, their manuscripts often do not meet the criteria for publication.

After having read so many manuscripts which were perfect examples of "how not to write for publication," I came upon the idea of writing this book. My suggestions and approach to writing for publication are the outgrowth of my experience as a clinician, academician, author and journal reviewer of manuscripts written by health professionals. By using a "how to approach," this book explains the fundamentals of writing for publication and encourages the reader to become not just a writer, but a published author. Through the use of examples particularized to the health professions, this text provides the aspiring writer with an instructional tool for learning how to write a journal or book-length manuscript that has a greater potential for being published.

The book is organized into five chapters. The first chapter introduces the reader to the subject of writing for publication. The topics covered include the five w's of writing a journal publication; the general criteria for acceptable journal manuscripts; the writing process; the qualities of a health professional writer and some do's and don'ts of writing for publication.

The second chapter identifies the principle components of a journal publication. The purpose and general characteristics of each of these elements are described. Suggestions on how to write each component are presented.

The third chapter describes ten types of journal publications which the health professional would most likely be interested in learning how to write. The primary goal and characteristics of each of these types of publications are explained. As a guideline to learning how to write such manuscripts, examples of published articles and the review criteria used by some journals are presented.

Chapter four introduces the health professional to the subject of book writing. It begins with the five w's of writing a book publication. This is followed by an account of my personal trials and tribulations of book writing; suggestions on how to approach a publisher; and points to consider in a publisher-author agreement.

The fifth and final chapter offers advice on how to start and finish writing the manuscript. It also presents ten basic steps to writing for publication and explains how to get into print.

At the end of each chapter, there is a series of questions and answers that are directed toward the topics covered. In order for the reader to acquire more information on a particular subject, a list of references and suggested readings is provided at the end of each chapter rather than at the end of the book as is customary. In this way, the reader can progress to more technical or theoretical knowledge before going on to the next chapter.

Although I have used a "how to approach," this book does not propose that all manuscripts can or should be written in precisely the same manner. Writing is a creative activity in that one's knowledge and expertise is reflected in the content and one's personality is brought forward in the style of writing. Even if certain guidelines and rules must be observed in writing for publication, the health professional writer can and should produce a work that is original, new and worthwhile.

The publication of this book could not have been possible without the assistance and support of certain institutions and persons. I wish to express my gratitude to the Université de Montréal, for giving me the time for writing this book during my sabbatical year; to the Faculty of

Medicine, Université de Montréal, for their financial support; to the Canadian Occupational Therapy Foundation, for awarding me a publications grant; to Charles C Thomas Publishers, for providing me with the opportunity of getting published; to La corporation professionnelle des ergothérapeutes du Québec ("Professional Corporation of Occupational Therapists of Quebec"), for encouraging me to write this book; and to the following journals, for granting me permission to reprint their material: *American Journal of Occupational Therapy, Archives of Physical Medicine and Rehabilitation, Canadian Journal of Occupational Therapy, Journal of Allied Health, Journal of Nursing Administration and Nurse Educator, Physical Therapy,* and *Rehabilitation Nursing.* A very special thanks to Geraldine Moore, who offered valuable suggestions for improving the content, and to Johanne Viau, who typed the final manuscript for this book.

Last but not least, I wish to acknowledge my husband, Chris for his continuous support, encouragement, and guidance in bringing this book to fruition; I owe him more than words can express.

CONTENTS

THE
HEALTH PROFESSIONAL'S GUIDE
TO
WRITING FOR PUBLICATION

Chapter I

WRITING FOR PUBLICATION

If you do not write for publication there is little point in writing at all.
George Bernard Shaw

For some health professionals, writing for publication is viewed as a challenging, exciting and worthwhile experience which merits repetition. Yet, for others, it is regarded as a time-consuming, laborious and frustrating endeavor, never to be undertaken again. Why the difference of viewpoints?

One possible explanation is that health professionals who know how to write for publication, consider writing in a positive light, while those who do not know how, view it negatively. All health professionals can write, however, writing for publication is a skill that is acquired and developed through a clear understanding and ability to apply certain writing principles. For this purpose, let us begin at the beginning, and introduce the subject of writing for publication.

The topics covered in this chapter include the five w's of writing a journal publication; the general criteria for acceptable journal manuscripts; the writing process; the qualities of a health professional writer; and some do's and don'ts of writing for publication. Although this chapter focuses on writing a journal publication, many of the principles presented can also be applied to a book publication.

FIVE W'S OF WRITING A JOURNAL PUBLICATION
WHAT? WHO? WHY? WHERE? WHEN?

One of the best ways to learn about any subject, is to ask the right questions, to search for the answers, and to think about the answers. By asking and answering five basic questions, this section introduces the subject of writing a journal publication and encourages the reader to reflect upon the issues presented.

What is a Journal Publication?

In this book, a journal publication is defined as an original paper which (a) is written by a health professional, for health professionals, (b) is published in a peer-reviewed journal, and (c) contributes to the advancement of knowledge and practice in the field of health science. A journal publication can be one of several types. It can be written in the form of a feature or full-length article (e.g., research or theoretical article); a brief report (e.g., case or clinical report); a book review or a letter to the editor. Thus, in this book, a journal publication does not refer only to research articles, but rather includes all papers which are published in a peer-reviewed journal whose purpose and scope is designed for health professionals.

Who Can Write a Journal Publication?

Health professionals who have ideas, experiences or knowledge that may be of value and interest to their colleagues in the field of health science can write a journal publication. Whether you practice as a clinician, a consultant, an educator, a researcher or an administrator, you can become a health professional writer and contribute to the advancement of your career and your profession.

Why Write or Read a Journal Publication?

There are several reasons why health professionals should write a journal publication:

1. To develop, disseminate and share scientifically valid and clinically meaningful information.
2. To contribute to the body of knowledge in the field of health science.
3. To promote the maximum quality of health care.
4. To stimulate further research.

From the reader's perspective, a journal publication encourages the health professional:

1. To critically review and assess the author's findings, observations and opinions.

2. To apply reported theoretical or clinical knowledge in a wide variety of settings.
3. To provide the most up-to-date assessment and treatment interventions.

Where Are Journal Manuscripts Published?

There is a plethora of journals which publish papers contributing to the advancement of knowledge and practice in the field of health science. Stein (1984) reports that there are over 6,000 journals that are related to health research. Because of this enormous number, health professional writers have a wide choice of journals to which their manuscripts can be submitted. Appendix A presents a list of some 100 journals in the health field.

Depending upon the reading audience for whom your paper is intended, you can select the journal which would be most appropriate for your work. For example, if you are a nurse, you may consider writing a paper for other American nurses (e.g., *American Journal of Nursing*), or for nurses in another country (e.g., *Canadian Nurse*). On the other hand, rather than address your peers, you may want to impart information to occupational therapists (e.g., *American Journal of Occupational Therapy*), or to a specific group of social workers (e.g., *Journal of Gerontological Social Work*). In determining your reading audience, you will also be able to write in a style that can be understood by the readers.

When Should You Write a Journal Publication?

There is no better time for preparing a journal publication than "write" now. If you have developed a new assessment or treatment approach, or if you have reviewed past knowledge in a new and different perspective, or if you have conducted a research study, it is recommended that you communicate in writing this knowledge as soon as possible. Waiting a year or two before writing your paper, may result in the information being outdated by the time it is published. By writing your paper today, you can promote tomorrow's development and advancement of the body of knowledge in the field of health science.

GENERAL CRITERIA FOR
ACCEPTABLE JOURNAL MANUSCRIPTS

In most health professional journals, a manuscript submitted for publication is subjected to a critical peer review by two or three journal reviewers. These reviewers are either members of the journal's editorial (or review) board or are ad hoc consultants who have a specific expertise in a particular subject (Cleather, 1981). When a manuscript is submitted for review, the editor selects the journal reviewers who are most qualified to review the work. Generally, the identities of the reviewers and the author of the manuscript are not revealed to each other and consequently, the evaluation is a blind peer review.

It is the role and responsibility of the journal reviewer to objectively evaluate a manuscript's quality and appropriateness for publication, and to recommend to the editor whether the paper is suitable or not for publication. In this way, the review process serves to assist the editor in selecting the papers best suited for the journal's readership (Cleather, 1981). The editor makes the final decision and advises the author of the outcome of the blind peer review.

The criteria used to evaluate a manuscript's quality and suitability for publication, are determined by the individual journal. Since there are no standardized criteria which are used by all health professional journals, the criteria can vary from one journal to the next. In general, however, when assessing a manuscript's suitability for publication, the journal reviewer examines its quality and overall value in terms of the content and the writing style.

Content

The content of a journal publication refers to the significance or meaning of the written information. In most health professional journals, the principle content areas include research, practice, administration and education. The quality of a manuscript's content is assessed with regards to the following elements:

Relevance and Appropriateness of the Topic

Does the topic meet the aims and scope of the journal? Is the subject matter of interest to the journal's readership?

Originality of the Work

Does the content duplicate material recently published elsewhere? Are the author's own analysis and findings reported? Does the content reflect a new approach to a previously published subject?

Potential Contribution of the Work

If published, will the paper contribute to the advancement of knowledge and practice in the health field? Will it be of value to a specific health discipline or to the health field in general?

Writing Style

Good writing style is of paramount importance for all publications. No matter how good and appropriate a manuscript's content may be, if the writing style is poor, it will be considered unsuitable for publication. For a manuscript to qualify for journal publication, it must be logically organized and use precise and concise language.

Logical Organization

The health professional embarking on the journey of writing a journal publication must organize the paper into a logical sequence of facts, events, thoughts and ideas. In its most basic form, the paper is divided into three main parts: (a) the beginning (title, abstract, introduction), (b) the main body of text, and (c) the end (conclusion, acknowledgments, references). Depending upon the type of publication, the parts which constitute the main body of text will vary.

There should be a logical progression of thought from one part of the paper to the next, from one paragraph to the next and from one sentence to the next. According to Morgan (1984), well-organized paragraphs are the key to a clear and logical organization of the paper. Within each paragraph, there should be a logical and organized development of the subject, thereby contributing to the overall flow of thought in the paper. A smooth and clear transition from one paragraph to the next will lead to clear writing and coherent reading.

Precise and Concise Language

A well-written journal publication is one that is precise in its use and choice of words. Very often, the novice writer does not accord enough attention to choosing the most accurate and appropriate words, expressions or terms. This results in the reader having difficulty understanding exactly what the author intends to communicate. Perhaps the words used are clear to the writer but they are confusing, ambiguous or unclear to the reader. Since the author writes for the reader, every attempt should be made to be as precise as possible.

In general, you should try to avoid the use of scholarly, technical or professional terminology that would not be understood by the reader. Instead, use words which are exact, accurate and clearly defined. Vague and general terms that denote doubt or uncertainty should be replaced with specific, distinct and definite words. The tone of the paper should be neutral and impersonal; use objective rather than subjective words and terms.

It is important to remember that in writing a journal publication, once you have defined a term, concept or variable in a particular way, it is not acceptable to casually replace it with words that have the same or nearly the same meaning or significance (Wilson, 1985). For example, in describing a multidisciplinary approach to treating the non-oral person, one should not substitute "transdisciplinary" or "interdisciplinary" for the term "multidisciplinary," unless you have defined them as meaning the exact same thing. This principle also applies in replacing "non-oral" with "non-communicative," "non-verbal," or "non-vocal." Although these terms may often be used interchangeably in speech, they do not mean the exact same thing and should not be used as such in writing, unless otherwise specified.

In a recent editorial of the *Canadian Journal of Rehabilitation,* Vargo (1987) addresses the issue of terminology in relation to disability. He points out to health care professionals that the language we use to describe people with disabilities can implicitly or explicitly portray these persons as stereotypes, overemphasize the negative effects of disability and deny them the individuality, dignity and respect that is rightfully theirs. It is therefore crucial that words be carefully chosen when writing about people with disabilities.

In light of this issue, Vargo (1987) and the editorial board of the *Canadian Journal of Rehabilitation* recommend that authors submitting manuscripts to this journal should:

1. Avoid terms which deny individuals with disabilities of their dignity and respect; e.g., "cripples," "victims," or "cases."

2. Avoid terms which reduce individuals to medical conditions; e.g.,

"paraplegics," or "epileptics." Similarly, rather than referring to "the handicapped" or "the disabled," speak in terms of "individuals who are handicapped" or "people with disabilities."

3. Refrain from using terms which focus on the negative effects of disability; e.g., "confined to a wheelchair," or "afflicted with . . . " Use instead "wheelchair user" or "the person has . . . "

Concise writing in a journal publication is characterized by text which is brief, succinct and comprehensive. It is important that the writer avoid superfluous detail and verbose text. Each sentence and paragraph should be relevant and essential. A paper which fails to use concise language results in a long and boring text, and interferes with its readability. The end result is that the reader becomes frustrated and loses interest in the paper.

To illustrate one journal's general criteria for acceptable manuscripts, that of *Physical Therapy* is presented in Table 1. *Physical Therapy* is an official publication of the American Physical Therapy Association. All manuscripts submitted to this journal are reviewed in terms of the following criteria: communication ability, use of language, organization, title, references, figures and tables, and acknowledgments. Depending upon the type of manuscript being reviewed, this journal uses additional and more specific criteria (see "Feature Articles" and "Brief Reports" in Chap. III).

With reference to general criteria for acceptable manuscripts, the ten most frequent stylistic and grammatical problems that I have encountered as a journal reviewer, include the following:

1. Text is written in note form rather than as a narrative text.
2. Acronyms and abbreviations are used without having been firstly written in full.
3. Inconsistent expression of numbers and numerals is used.
4. Text is overloaded with reference citations, direct quotations, and tables or figures which make for difficult reading.
5. Typographical, grammatical, spelling and punctuation errors are present.
6. Inconsistent mixing of tenses, redundancies and poor syntax appear in the text.
7. Names of medical conditions (e.g., cerebral palsy), professions (e.g., physical therapy) and professionals (e.g., physical therapists), are capitalized when they should not be.

TABLE I
GENERAL CRITERIA FOR ACCEPTABLE MANUSCRIPTS:
PHYSICAL THERAPY

FOR ALL TYPES OF MANUSCRIPTS

A.   COMMUNICATION ABILITY:

Clear, precise expression (e.g., not vague, ambiguous, obscure)
Concise expression
Presentation of ideas: • Logical sequence
                       • Understandable relationship of ideas
                       • Smooth flow between ideas

B.   USE OF LANGUAGE

Correct grammar
Acceptable, professional terminology (e.g., no jargon, eponyms, slang, or stilted terms)
Current scientific vocabulary (to rule out archaic but acceptable words)
Abbreviations representative of current scientific literature (including those in text, figures, and tables)
Consistent style throughout
Concepts within each paper consistently directed to same educational level of particular group of readers (including physical therapist assistant)
Objectives and nonthreatening approach in communication (to rule out inflammatory, derogatory, or biased comments)

C.   ORGANIZATION

Appropriate sections and subsections included according to the type of manuscript
Logical sequence of content
Correct placement of content in sections or subsections
Consistent order of presenting similar factors in different sections

D.   TITLE

Descriptive of topic as presented in text
Briefly presented

E.   REFERENCES

Relevant documentation as supportive rationale for specific factors (not just relevant to general topics)
Logical interpretation of concepts advocated by resources
Recent sources included
Accurately presented according to APTA Style Manual
Satisfactory in number (not too few to support rationale or too many on same point)

TABLE I (continued)

FOR ALL TYPES OF MANUSCRIPTS

F.   FIGURES/TABLES

Cited in text
Cited in sequential order
Complement text (not duplicate)
Clarify content of text
Satisfactory in number (no need for more or less to be used)
Content agrees with text
Adequate detail to have figures and legends, tables and titles, and appendixes stand
    alone (not too little or too much)
Visually clear pertinent details
Accurate titles and legends
Figure legends understandable without reading text
Tables presented in accordance with APTA Style Manual
Abbreviations in accordance with APTA Style Manual
Abbreviations consistent with text
Photo consent included as needed
Permission to reprint included as needed

G.   ACKNOWLEDGMENTS

Presented in accordance with APTA Style Manual

Reprinted from Physical Therapy Criteria Packet Review Forms, with the permission of the American Physical Therapy Association.

8. Sexist rather than nonsexist language has been used.
9. References in the reference list are not presented in conformance with the journal's guidelines or do not have a corresponding citation in the text.
10. Citations in the text are not presented according to the journal's guidelines, or do not have a corresponding reference in the reference list.

THE WRITING PROCESS

There are three stages inherent in the writing process: planning, writing and rewriting.

Stage I: Planning

Before beginning to write, you need to identify a working plan of action; you must plan your work. This means primarily planning your writing and planning your time.

Planning your Writing

Planning your writing essentially involves two important activities: preparing an outline and gathering of information.

Preparing an Outline: A well-drawn outline serves to establish the framework and direction of your paper. According to Schlosberg (1986), organized writing demands an outline. This author compares writing without an outline to riding a horse with no saddle; at first it is exciting, but you are bound to fall off sooner or later. An outline keeps your writing on track.

As illustrated in Table II, a basic or initial outline should include the following elements:

1. Subject: What is the subject or topic of the paper? Would it be of interest and value to health professionals? Has a paper on the same or similar topic ever been published?
2. Working title: What are one or two possible titles for the paper?
3. Reading audience: For whom are you writing your manuscript? Do you wish to address your peers or do you intend to write for other health professionals?
4. Journals: Which journals are you considering for review and publication of your manuscript?
5. Type of publication: Which type of journal publication are you planning to write?
6. Purpose: What is the purpose of your paper?
7. Component parts: How will you divide the manuscript into its component parts? What headings and sub-headings would be most appropriate for these divisions?

This initial outline serves as the basis for beginning a manuscript. In essence, it is a working outline in that it will be further developed and expanded throughout the writing process.

Gathering of Information: Once you have prepared your initial outline, it is necessary that you gather the information you will need for writing. That is, all resources such as journal publications, books, reference lists, conference reports, patient records or data which will serve as your

TABLE II
INITIAL OUTLINE OF A JOURNAL MANUSCRIPT

Subject

Drooling in cerebral palsy

Working Title

The relationship between drooling and seating position in children with cerebral palsy

Reading Audience

Occupational therapists

Journals

American Journal of Occupational Therapy
Canadian Journal of Occupational Therapy, or
Physical and Occupational Therapy in Pediatrics

Type of Publication

Feature, research article

Purpose

To report to occupational therapists the findings of a research study which examined the relationship between drooling and seating position in children with cerebral palsy.

Component Parts

Abstract
Introduction
Body of text: Literature review
   • Drooling
   • Cerebral palsy
   Methodology
   • Subjects
   • Measuring instruments
   • Procedure
   • Data analysis
   Results
   Discussion
Conclusion
Acknowledgments
References

source of information should be identified and be made accessible for you to use. This information then needs to be categorized and organized according to the elements identified in your outline.

Planning your Time

In order to write a maximum quality paper with a minimum waste of time and effort, it is necessary to identify a realistic writing schedule. Some authors prefer to schedule intense, regular periods of writing (e.g., six to ten hours each day), while others adopt shorter and more irregular writing schedules (e.g., two to three hours per day, one or two days per week). After you have prepared your initial outline, estimate the amount of time you will need to write each of the components of your manuscript, by determining the frequency and duration of your writing periods.

It is almost impossible to suggest how much time will be required for you to prepare and write a journal manuscript because there are several important factors which need to be considered:

Writing Skills and Experience of the Author: If this is your first attempt at writing for publication, you will require more time to develop and improve your writing skills than the experienced writer. The quality of your writing is influenced by your writing experience; the more you write, the better writer you will become.

Number of Authors Writing the Manuscript: Whether you are the sole author or whether you are writing with one or more authors is an important factor to consider in planning your time. For the sole author, whose writing skills and experience have yet to be acquired and developed, writing can be a very slow, difficult and solitary activity. Much time can be saved by reading and studying the writing styles of published papers. It is also recommended that you consult with an experienced writer who can offer you some advice or feedback on your manuscript.

Writing in collaboration with one or more experienced authors may be a worthwhile alternative for the novice writer. Multiple authorship can be advantageous in that there is (a) a division of labor among authors, (b) peer assistance and constructive criticism, (c) mutual support and encouragement, and (d) sharing of ideas, experiences and knowledge. There are however, disadvantages related to multiple authorship. These include such problems as differing writing styles and abilities among authors, personality differences and issues of authorship credit, power and control (Nehring & Durham, 1986).

Type of Publication: Depending upon the type of publication selected, some manuscripts require more time to write than others. For example, a book requires more time to write than a journal publication. Similarly, a feature article involves a greater investment of time than does a brief report or a book review. It is important that you consider this factor in your time plan.

Stage 2: Writing

After you have planned your work, it is time to work your plan; you can begin writing. The actual act of putting your thoughts into words and communicating these words onto paper, can at times be difficult and demanding. It is important that you select the writing instrument that is best for you; whether you use a pen and paper, a manual or electric typewriter, or a word processor, is a matter of personal preference.

Although there is no right or wrong way to begin writing, it is suggested that you use your outline to direct you in organizing your writing. Some writers prefer to follow the order of the elements identified in their outline and as such, begin with the introduction and proceed according to the plan, until ending with the references. Others, on the other hand, feel more productive or creative by beginning with that section of the paper which generates the most ideas or that which appears to be the easiest to write. Regardless of which approach you choose, do not at this time be too concerned about your writing style. Simply use your outline as your guide and write your thoughts as they come to you. It is in the rewriting stage that you will have the opportunity of editing your paper.

Stage 3: Rewriting

The purpose of rewriting is primarily to improve the manuscript's quality in terms of its content and writing style. The rewriting stage permits you to:

1. Improve the syntax and organization of the manuscript.
2. Correct any important errors or omissions of information.
3. Delete any repetitions of facts or redundancies.
4. Assure that the choice of words is precise and concise.
5. Correct typographical, grammatical, spelling and punctuation errors.

6. Check for accuracy of citations, quotations, numerical data, tables, figures and references.
7. Verify that the manuscript conforms to the journal's editorial style, as specified in their guidelines.

Rewriting of the manuscript will require that you produce multiple drafts until it is ready to be submitted for review. According to Bishop (1981), even experienced writers must prepare several drafts for the purpose of obtaining a "polished" manuscript. You should stop rewriting when you feel that your manuscript has potential for being published. Evaluate your work critically and rewrite, until it is just "write."

QUALITIES OF A HEALTH PROFESSIONAL WRITER

As a health professional, you already possess certain qualities that are essential to writing for publication. You are a good problem solver, an organized thinker and a professional with clinical knowledge, skills and experience (Duffy & Philbrick, 1985). In addition to these professional competencies, there are other qualities which either need to be acquired or further developed in order to become a published author. These include:

1. Perseverance: The health professional writer needs to be able to persevere in the writing process, in spite of opposition, discouragement or obstacles. There will always be certain factors which may temporarily deter you from writing, but perseverance in a time-consuming activity such as writing for publication is an essential quality for the published author-to-be.

2. Self-discipline: Writing for publication requires self-discipline. This implies that you must impose upon yourself a certain structure and course of action for writing. It is very difficult, if not impossible, to become a writer if you are not disciplined in your thoughts and actions.

3. Unbiased attitude: As a health professional writer, you need to display in your writing, an objective, unbiased and impartial attitude. Just as you are diplomatic and tactful in your professional relations with others, so must you be in your writing. The tone of your paper should reflect the professional and unbiased attitude you are expected to demonstrate in your clinical practice.

4. Motivation: One cannot become a writer, if one does not have the desire, the determination and the motivation to write. Each health profes-

sional has his or her own personal reasons for aspiring to become a published author. Whether your reason be for career promotion or simply for the pleasure of writing and the satisfaction of seeing your name in print, is not of critical importance. What is significant, is that your reason be strong enough to provide you with the impetus to write successfully for publication.

DO'S AND DON'TS OF WRITING FOR PUBLICATION

In writing for publication, it is just as essential to know what not to do, as it is to know what to do. The following are important do's and don'ts of writing for publication:

1. Do select a relevant subject: It is important to select a subject which will be of interest and value to the intended reading audience of health professionals. Very often, the timeliness of your paper will be closely related to the relevance of the subject matter; if your work addresses an issue which is of current interest and importance, its potential for getting published will be enhanced.

2. Do choose an appropriate writing environment: Writing for publication requires much concentration, especially for the novice writer. It is therefore advisable that you write in an environment propitious to good concentration. Only you can identify the setting which enables you to write your best.

3. Do write for the reader: Writing involves communication of meaningful information between the writer and the reader. For this reason, you must write for the reader and not for yourself. This requires that you write at the reader's level by using the appropriate language, detail and style of writing.

4. Do develop and improve your writing skills: Writing is an acquired skill that requires constant, long-term practice (Bishop, 1981). Your writing skills can be developed and improved by consulting various reference books, the most important of which is the dictionary. Different dictionaries provide different entries and definitions and for this reason, it is advisable to use more than one. It is also recommended that you read recent works in the journal you intend to approach in order to examine the types of papers that journal publishes and the writing styles of these publications. Read these works as a writer, and not just as a reader. Use them as a model for learning how to write for publication. In addition, having your paper read by an experienced writer can provide

you with valuable feedback with regards to the strengths and weaknesses of your writing.

5. Do focus on success, not failure: A positive attitude towards writing is a must for all authors. If you feel that what you have to say is not important or if you think that your manuscript does not merit publication, then you will probably never see your paper in print. On the other hand, by being confident in your ability to write and proud of the quality of your work, your chances of success will be better assured.

6. Do not begin writing without first planning your work: The planning stage of the writing process is the key to successful writing. Although this may seem self-evident, it is not obvious to many health professionals who are new writers and consequently, much time and effort is wasted. Just as you plan your assessment and treatment interventions with your clients, so must you premeditate your writing. It is only then, that you will be able to yield the maximum quality of your efforts.

7. Do not expect your first draft to be your last: There will be several drafts of your manuscript until it is ready to be submitted for review. Each part of your paper will require rewriting so as to improve the content and the writing style. In reality, your first draft is only a canvas in that it serves as the background or base of your final manuscript.

8. Do not be disappointed if your submitted manuscript requires revision: Even your submitted manuscript may be subjected to further rewriting following the outcome of the journal's peer review. A large number of manuscripts I have reviewed were accepted, conditional upon minor or moderate revisions. This type of recommendation implies that the paper will be published, provided that the author rewrite and improve certain parts of the paper in accordance with the journal reviewers' comments. As this is so often the case, do not be disappointed because in reality, your revision of the paper will most probably result in its being published.

QUESTIONS? ANSWERS

Question

As a clinician, I am expected primarily to treat clients and consequently, my hospital administration does not allow me to take time from my work to write for publication. How can I explain to the management the merits and need for my writing a journal publication?

Answer

For clinicians, one of the most frequent barriers to writing for publication is the lack of time available for writing. It is recommended that you obtain the administration's support and approval of your writing project by explaining the merits and need for your paper and perhaps then, you will be allowed to allocate some work time for writing.

Signify to the management the importance of communicating and sharing knowledge through a journal publication. Also, indicate that the name of the center or institution will be acknowledged in the publication and that health professionals reading it will recognize the work conducted at your setting. Even if you are permitted to use a certain amount of work time for writing your paper, be prepared to invest some of your own time as well.

Question

What are some of the emotional barriers which may prevent the health professional from writing for publication?

Answer

The emotional barriers of writing for publication are not confined to health professionals alone, but rather can be encountered by any writer. These include (a) fear of rejection of the manuscript, (b) lack of confidence in one's ability to write, (c) fear of criticism from one's peers, (d) writer's anxiety/block, and (e) a sense of being overwhelmed by the size of the writing project.

Question

Why is it advisable that I determine the intended reading audience before I begin to write my paper?

Answer

By identifying your reading audience before you begin to write, you will be able to write in a style that can be understood by the readers. For example, suppose you are an occupational therapist and the topic of your paper is the role of the occupational therapist in the prosthetic training of persons with upper limb amputations. Will your reading audience be occupational therapists, physical therapists, nurses or prosthetists? The paper's content and writing style for this topic will not be the same for each of these health professionals. If you are addressing your peers, it will not be necessary to define those terms that are familiar to occupational therapists. On the other hand, if you are writing for other health professionals, then many of these same terms will need to be defined.

By determining your targeted reading audience from the onset, you will also be able to select the most appropriate journal to which your manuscript will be submitted for review and publication.

Question

I would like to write a journal publication in collaboration with one or more authors. When and how do we determine the order of the authors' names on our publication?

Answer

Before even beginning to write the paper, it is advisable that the authors determine the order of their names so as to avoid any problems of group conflict and authorship credit. There are basically three ways in which this can be decided.

Firstly, the names can be placed in alphabetical order, however, this method does not necessarily recognize the author who was the principle writer or leader of the group. Secondly, the authors' names can be identified according to each person's degree of writing participation; the person who was the principle writer will be firstly acknowledged and the individual who did the least writing will be the last to be identified. Thirdly, if the situation is such that there was an equal division of writing among the authors, then the group of writers may decide that for this particular paper the order will be randomly determined. For future publications as a group however, the order of the authors' names would be alternated so as to provide each writer with the opportunity of being the first author at some time.

REFERENCES AND SUGGESTED READINGS

References

Bishop, B. (1981). Contents of a paper for presentation. *Physiotherapy Canada, 33,* 277–280.

Cleather, J. (1981). Manuscript review and the editing process. *Physiotherapy Canada, 33,* 283–286.

Duffy, K. L., & Philbrick, M. S. (1985). Give publishing a try: Step-by-step guidelines for would-be writers. *AORN Journal, 42,* 230–234.

Morgan, P. P. (1984). To write better paragraphs. *Canadian Medical Association Journal, 130,* 1255.

Nehring, W., & Durham, J. D. (1986). Multiple authorship and professional advancement. *Dimensions of Critical Care Nursing, 5,* 58–62.

Schlosberg, J. (1986, July). The writer's organizational toolbox. *Writer's Digest,* pp. 25–27.

Stein, F. (1984). *Anatomy of research in allied health* (2nd ed.). Cambridge, MA: Schenkman.

Vargo, J. W. (1987). What's in a name? A note on terminology. *Canadian Journal of Rehabilitation, 1,* 75–76.

Wilson, H. S. (1985). Disseminating research: The scholar's commitment. *Journal of Nursing Administration, 15,* 6–8.

Suggested Readings

Acquaviva, F. A., & Malone, R. A. (1981). *The power of positive persuasion: A professional's guide to communications.* Laurel, MD: RAMSCO.

Delton, J. (1985). *The 29 most common writing mistakes & how to avoid them.* Cincinnati, OH: Writer's Digest Books.

King, L. S. (1978). *Why not say it clearly: A guide to scientific writing.* Boston: Little, Brown.

Shertzer, M. (1986). *The elements of grammar.* New York: Macmillan.

Strunk, W., Jr., & White, E. B. (1979). *Elements of style* (3rd ed.). New York: Macmillan.

Turabian, K. L. (1973). *A manual for writers of term papers, theses, and dissertations* (4th ed.). Chicago: University of Chicago Press.

Willeford, G., Jr. (1987). *Webster's new world medical word finder* (4th ed.). New York: Prentice Hall.

Woolley, A. S., & Hatcher, B. J. (1986). Teaching students to write for publication. *Journal of Nursing Education, 25,* 300–301.

Zinsser, W. (1980). *On writing well: An informal guide to writing nonfiction* (2nd ed.). New York: Harper & Row.

Chapter II

COMPONENT PARTS
OF A JOURNAL PUBLICATION

Reading maketh a full man; conference a ready man; and writing an exact man.

Francis Bacon

A journal publication is composed of several component parts, all of which are inter-related and contribute to the quality and value of the manuscript as a whole. Figure 1 presents the principle components of a journal publication to be discussed in this chapter, as well as the order in which they are usually presented. It is important to note that not all journal publications include all of these components; depending upon the type of publication selected, there is variability in the parts which constitute the paper. In addition, not every component is identified as such with a heading, but yet the publication can incorporate that component; depending upon the editorial style adopted by the journal, the use of headings and sub-headings will vary.

Since each journal has its own guidelines to preparing a manuscript for publication, it is possible that a journal's specifications or requirements might differ slightly from some of the material presented in this chapter. Thus, it is strongly recommended that you read and conform to the rules and/or guidelines of the journal to which your manuscript will be submitted and bear in mind that the information presented here is not the final word on the subject.

TITLE

The purpose of the title of a journal publication is to identify the subject matter of the paper and to attract the intended reading audience. The title is the first and most frequently read component of a journal publication. A large number of persons read the title without necessarily reading the paper mainly because the title is published in various

23

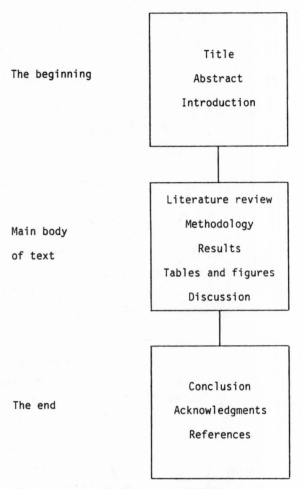

Figure 1. Component parts of a journal publication.

resources: the journal's table of contents; periodical indexes and abstracts; bibliographies and reference lists. Generally, after examining the title, the reader decides whether or not to read the paper. This is why it is important to write an appropriate title; that is, one that reflects the paper's content, attracts the intended reading audience and uses clear and precise words.

Types of Titles

Rather than classifying titles as being either short or long, it is perhaps more useful to group them according to the degree of specificity of the subject matter and the size of the intended reading audience (see Table III). Most titles of health journal publications can be categorized as being one of four types. By examining the titles of several published articles, the characteristics of each of these types of titles will be described. It is important to note that my comments on these titles are based upon the information provided in the bibliographic reference alone. Reading the publication in its entirety would be necessary to verify these observations.

TABLE III
FOUR TYPES OF TITLES

	Specificity of Subject Matter	*Size of Reading Audience*
Type 1	very general	large reading audience of health professionals
Type 2	specific	large reading audience of health professionals
Type 3	specific	large reading audience within a particular health profession
Type 4	highly specialized	specific reading audience within a particular health profession

Type 1 Title

A type 1 title is one that reflects a broad or very general subject which appeals to a large reading audience of health professionals. The following is an example of a type 1 title:

Cook, H. L., Beery, M., Sauter, S. V. H., & DeVellis, R. F. (1987). Continuing education for health professionals. *American Journal of Occupational Therapy, 41,* 652–657.

Based on the title, it is likely that any health professional interested in continuing education might want to read this article. The fact that the paper was published in the *American Journal of Occupational Therapy* indicates that occupational therapists are one of the target reading audiences of health professionals. Also, since it is a multiple-authored paper, addressing a general subject, there is a strong possibility that the authors are not of the same discipline and that the paper provides a multidisciplinary perspective.

Type 2 Title

The type 2 title addresses a specific subject matter that would be of interest to a large reading audience of health professionals. An example of a type 2 title appears below:

Wilgosh, L. R., & Skaret, D. (1987). Employer attitudes toward hiring individuals with disabilities: A review of the recent literature. *Canadian Journal of Rehabilitation, 1,* 89–98.

The title of this article reveals to the reader the parameter studied (i.e., employer attitudes), the target population (i.e., individuals with disabilities), as well as the type of journal publication (i.e., review article). Since the paper was published in the *Canadian Journal of Rehabilitation,* it would probably appeal to any health professional interested in this specific subject. Thus, this kind of title is similar to the type 1 title in that it appeals to a large reading audience of health professionals, but differs in that the subject matter is more specific.

Type 3 Title

The third type of title is one that reveals a specific subject matter and is written for a large reading audience within a particular health profession. The following is an example of a type 3 title:

Tomlinson, A., & Williams, A. (1985). Communication skills in nursing: A practical account. *Nursing, 2,* 1121–1123.

From this title, it appears likely that any nurse, interested in the subject of communication skills, might be attracted to this paper. Although the subject is relatively specific and the intended reading audience is that of a particular health profession, a large number of these professionals are most apt to read this paper. Thus, the type 3 title differs from the other two kinds of titles in that it reflects a specific subject matter that would primarily be of interest to professionals of a specific health discipline. One cannot however, eliminate the possibility that this article might be worthwhile reading for health professionals who are not nurses.

Type 4 Title

The fourth type of title is one that identifies a highly specialized subject and that is intended for a specific audience of readers within a particular health profession. An example of a type 4 title is given below:

Weaver, S. A., Lange, L. R., & Vogts, V. M., (1988). Comparison of myoelectric and conventional prostheses for adolescent amputees. *American Journal of Occupational Therapy, 42,* 87–91.

In this example, the title designates a highly specialized subject that would be of interest primarily to occupational therapists involved in prosthetic training of adolescents with upper limb amputations. Thus, this type of title reflects a very distinct content area that is largely intended for a limited audience of readers within a particular health discipline. Most research articles have a type 4 title, thereby indicating the specialized nature of the research study.

How to Write the Title

In order to write the most suitable title for your paper, it is suggested that you determine the degree of specificity of the subject matter and the size of the intended reading audience. This can be done by referring to the characteristics of the four types of titles, as described in the preceding section. Which type of title would best suit your manuscript?

Once you have selected the type of title, you can proceed to writing several working titles. To do this, begin with your own ideas for the title and then review the titles of articles which treat the same or similar subject. In this way, you may not only generate ideas for your title, but may also verify that your title is as original as possible. After you have written several drafts of your manuscript, examine your working titles and select the one that is most appropriate for your paper. Be sure that the final title is grammatically correct, clear, accurate and meaningful.

ABSTRACT

In a journal publication, the abstract is basically, an overview of the paper's content; it succinctly and clearly describes what is being examined in the paper. By reading the abstract, the reader knows what the paper is about and thus can quickly decide whether or not to read it in its entirety. In order to attract the reading audience for whom the paper is intended, it is of paramount importance that the abstract be well-written.

Some health professional journals request that an abstract be prepared for all manuscripts submitted for publication, whereas others specify that an abstract is only to be included if the manuscript is a feature or full-length article. In most journals, an abstract is characterized by the following five features:

1. It is does not exceed 150–200 words.
2. It is written in one or two paragraphs.
3. It contains no reference citations and no direct quotations.
4. It has no abbreviations or acronyms (unless first written in full).
5. It is typed on a separate sheet of paper, when submitted and is presented separate from the body of the text, when published.

Types of Abstracts

According to Day (1979), there are primarily two types of abstracts: informational and indicative. An informational abstract briefly states the problem examined, the method(s) used, the results obtained and the principle conclusion(s) reached. This type of abstract is usually used in a research article. The indicative abstract on the other hand, descriptively identifies the paper's content, thereby essentially serving as a narrative table of contents. It is generally used for review articles or conference reports. The indicative abstract, because of its descriptive nature, seldom serves as a substitute for the full paper, whereas the informational abstract, because of its substantive nature, can often replace the reading of the whole paper.

The following is an example of an informational abstract:

One of the major factors in the decreasing functional ability of patients with progressive systemic sclerosis is involvement of the patient's hands with secondary immobility and contractures. In a 2-month study of 19 patients, we assessed whether dynamic splinting could decrease proximal interphalangeal (PIP) flexion contractures. Of the eight patients who completed the study, one experienced a statistically significant improvement in PIP range of motion as a result of the splinting. There was no evidence that the use of the splints served to maintain PIP extension when compared with the control hand. (Seeger & Furst, 1987, p. 118)*

This example of an informational abstract is composed of four sentences (93 words). The first sentence states the problem investigated; the

---

* *Note.* From "Effects of splinting in the treatment of hand contractures in progressive systemic sclerosis" by M. W. Seeger and D. E. Furst, 1987, *American Journal of Occupational Therapy, 41,* 118–121. Copyright 1987 by the American Occupational Therapy Association, Inc. Reprinted with permission.

second, identifies the method used; the third, reports the results obtained; and the fourth, presents the conclusion drawn. In a very small number of words, the authors clearly and succinctly highlight the factual essence of the paper.

The following is an example of an indicative abstract:

This paper briefly outlines the characteristics of teams, and teamwork, the dynamics of teamwork, team development and the processes of teambuilding. It examines the strengths and shortcomings of this approach, when teambuilding should not be used. Some teamwork guidelines and elements of teambuilding are presented along with three strategies for conflict management. Strategies for team growth and future implications of teambuilding are explored. (Heming, 1988, p. 15)*

In this indicative abstract, the author descriptively outlines the paper's content. In very few words (63), the abstract provides enough information for the reader to know what is the basic content of the paper, and to decide whether or not to read it in its entirety.

How to Write the Abstract

It is best to write the abstract after you have written (and rewritten) the paper. The primary reason for this is that in order to present an overview of the paper's content, you must know beforehand what information is to be imparted. Begin first by identifying which type of abstract is appropriate for your manuscript. Then, depending upon your choice of abstract, compose a few sentences which outline the factual essence of the paper's content. Be sure that your abstract is characterized by the qualities described earlier and that it clearly, accurately, and briefly presents an overview of the paper's content.

INTRODUCTION

The introduction of any written work is simply the beginning of the paper. In a journal publication, the purpose of the introduction is to capture the reader's interest and to clearly introduce the subject being addressed. Although the introduction is not always labeled as such, it is presented after the abstract, and before the main body of the text (Kittredge,

---

* *Note.* From "The titanic triumvirate: Teams, teamwork and teambuilding" by D. Heming, 1988, *Canadian Journal of Occupational Therapy, 55,* 15–20. Reprinted with permission.

1985). Thus, the introduction serves as the preliminary part of the actual paper and sets into proper perspective what is about to follow.

According to Day (1979), in a scientific paper, a good introduction presents the nature and scope of the problem, reviews the pertinent literature, states the method used and the principle results obtained. Since Day (1979) uses the term "scientific paper" for an original research report, he is in other words saying that the introduction of a research article should include these four elements. However, depending upon the type of journal publication, the inclusion of all these elements in the introduction is not always necessary. For example, the introduction of a review article does not state the method used and the principle results obtained because this type of paper does not present a methodology and results section.

Regardless of the type of journal publication, there is however, one basic principle suggested for writing this part of the paper; the introduction should provide the reader with sufficient background information for understanding the purpose and content of the paper.

How to Write the Introduction

Like the title and abstract components of a journal publication, it is best to write the introduction after you have written (and rewritten) the paper. In order to clearly introduce the paper's content, you must know beforehand what information is to be communicated. Many health professional writers find it easier to write the introduction after having prepared the abstract. By using the abstract as the basis for writing the introduction, they develop and amplify it so as to introduce the paper to the reader and to inspire further reading.

Regardless of whether you write the introduction before or after the abstract, it is important to bear in mind that these two components differ and consequently, one should not be written as an exact duplicate of the other. The abstract is a brief overview of the paper's content and is limited to a maximum number of words (usually 150–200 words). The introduction on the other hand, describes in more detail the subject being examined and therefore, its length is somewhat longer than the abstract. In addition, definitions of terms, descriptions of published works and reference citations are presented in the introduction but are not included in the abstract.

LITERATURE REVIEW

The literature review is that part of a journal publication in which the author surveys relevant and recent literature on the subject being addressed. Basically, it is a synthesis of previous works which have examined the same or similar subject. The review combines diverse concepts, findings or observations into a coherent whole and serves to succinctly report the present state of knowledge on a particular subject.

Why is it necessary to present a literature review? By examining the literature, the author is able:

1. To determine the existing body of knowledge on a particular subject.
2. To review and evaluate relevant publications.
3. To justify the need for the study.
4. To ascertain the originality of the work.
5. To establish (in the discussion part of the paper) the relationship between the study's findings and those reported by other authors.

The length of the literature review section depends primarily upon two factors: (a) the type of publication, and (b) the number of works which exist on a particular subject and which warrant review. In a feature article (12–18 pages), the literature review is usually of a significant length (i.e., several pages), whereas in a brief report (3–6 pages), the literature review is relatively short (i.e., several paragraphs). In writing any kind of journal manuscript however, it is important to bear in mind that you cannot allege that no literature exists on your subject without having thoroughly examined the literature.

Based on my experience as a journal reviewer, I have found that many novice writers either do not include a literature review section in their manuscript, or if they do, they seem to have much difficulty writing this part of the paper. Why is it that many submitted journal manuscripts do not include a literature review? One possible reason for this is that many health professionals mistakenly think that a search of the literature is conducted only in a research study, and as such, assume that a literature review section is presented only in a research article. It is important to emphasize that searching the literature is necessary to establish the originality of any work, and therefore, other types of journal publications can and should include a literature review section. For example, a new ideas report or a clinical report should present a brief review of the literature. Why do many health professionals have difficulty writing this part of the paper? I believe that those who do not know how to search the literature, have trouble writing the literature review. In light of these two problems, this section will first examine how to prepare for writing the literature review and then will explain how to write this part of the paper.

How to Prepare for Writing the Literature Review

There are three basic steps which are suggested for acquiring and organizing the information needed for writing the literature review: (a) search the literature, (b) read and evaluate the literature, and (c) organize the information.

Step 1: Search the Literature

The purpose of searching the literature is to identify relevant literature which exists on a particular subject. A literature search can be very simple or very complex; it can be a narrow search or an exhaustive search. The complexity and extent of the literature search will depend upon the number of related works which exist on a subject and the type of search that is conducted. There are basically two types of literature searches; a manual search and a computer-based search.

A manual (or non-computerized) search of the literature refers to your locating "by hand" the relevant literature. By searching through various resources (e.g., books, current periodicals, review journals, abstract and indexing journals, bibliographic listings), you will uncover those works which investigated the same or similar subject you are addressing. Because this type of search can be very time-consuming, it is strongly recommended that you consult with a librarian to guide you in determining where and how to find the information you are seeking. To help you begin a manual search, consider the following four suggestions:

1. Identify the topics related to your subject: By determining the topics related to your subject, you will be able to limit the scope of your literature search. Draw up a list of topics which are relevant to your subject, and whenever possible, divide them into subtopics.

2. Search the periodical literature: Your search should not be confined to textbook sources alone, but rather should also include periodical literature. Learn to use various review, abstract and indexing journals to help you locate bibliographic sources of literature in medicine, rehabilitation and health care.

3. Begin with the most recent publications: Generally, the more recent publications provide the present state of knowledge on a particular subject. The bibliographic references presented in these works, will help you identify other publications which need to be examined.

4. Find a good review article: If you are fortunate enough to locate a review article closely related to your subject, your literature search will probably be much easier to conduct. This type of article not only presents an exhaustive review of the literature, but also provides a large number of references which can be consulted.

Unlike a manual search, a computer-based (or computerized) search accesses an automated bibliographic data bank via a terminal or computer. Appropriate key words or indexing terms are used to search the literature and the computer provides a printout of the bibliographic information needed to locate the relevant publications. Various referral sources are used in a computerized search and include:

1. Automated informational retrieval systems (e.g., Medical Literature Analysis and Retrieval System [MEDLARS], MEDLARS on Line [MEDLINE]).
2. Abstracting periodicals (e.g., *Excerpta Medica Abstract Journals, Psychological Abstracts, Dissertation Abstracts*).
3. Annual reviews (e.g., *Annual Review of Medicine*).
4. Indexing journals (e.g., *Index Medicus, Cumulative Index to Nursing and Allied Health Literature, Science Citation Index*).
5. Bibliographical Indexes (e.g., *Cumulated Index Medicus*).

If properly conducted, a computer-based search can be advantageous in that you can save much time and energy in identifying those works which are relevant to the subject being searched. For this purpose, it is strongly recommended that you consult with a librarian whose expertise will be indispensable for simplifying and maximizing the effectiveness of a computer-based search.

Once you have completed the search of the literature, you will have acquired a list of relevant references which should be consulted. Through library loans and photocopies, these publications can be made readily accessible for you to examine. Since the bibliographic reference does not provide sufficient information as to the relevance of the paper's content, it is suggested that you now proceed to reading and evaluating the literature you have identified.

Step 2: Read and Evaluate the Literature

The literature identified in Step 1 needs to be attentively read and evaluated to determine which publications are pertinent to the subject you are addressing. It is possible that after you read a study's abstract or the publication in its entirety, you discover that the content does not provide the information you are seeking or that you do not consider it valuable or appropriate. Thus, by reading and evaluating the literature, you will eliminate certain papers and select those works which provide you with information that you can use to write the literature review.

As you read through and evaluate each publication, it is important that you use a systematic and efficient method for recording and synthesizing the information. For this purpose, Cox and West (1982) recommend the use of 5″ × 8″ cards; for each publication, a file card is used to indicate the bibliographic information and to record the relevant information. In making your notes, consider the answers to the following questions:

- Why do you consider this paper to be relevant?
- What are the subtopics of the paper?
- Which components of the paper provide information that you can use in writing your literature review?
- Is the paper's literature review complete? Does it omit important writings? Does it provide you with useful information?
- How does the paper's content differ from other publications?
- Are the results the same or different? Are the methods the same or different?
- What are the strengths and weaknesses of the paper?
- Is it a recent or old publication? Is the information new and up-to-date or is it old and outdated?

Step 3: Organize the Information

After you have read and evaluated the literature, it is suggested that you organize the information you have obtained and recorded. By determining the subtopics of the literature review section of your manuscript, you can group or classify your file cards accordingly. For example, arrange your cards under such sub-headings as etiology, incidence, symptoms, assessment and treatment methods. After completing step 3, you can begin to write the literature review of your paper.

How to Write the Literature Review

As explained earlier, the literature review is a synthesis of previous works which have examined the same or similar subject. To begin writing this component of the paper, it is recommended that you take each of the subtopics (identified in Step 3) and in your own words, compose a narrative text which critically examines and reviews the relevant literature. Several versions of the literature review will be necessary to improve the content and writing style of the text.

In writing your review of the literature, it is critical that you identify the sources of your information by citing the works being reviewed; you must indicate to the reader from where the information originates. There are several ways to do this, however the three most frequently used methods of reference citations in the text are (a) the citation order system, (b) the alphabet-number system, and (c) the author-date system.

Citation Order System

The citation order system is basically a number system. The works cited are numbered consecutively, in the order in which they first appear in the text. The number appropriate to each work cited, corresponds to the same number used to list the reference at the end of the paper. In the text, the number assigned to each citation is placed at the appropriate point of the narrative, either in parentheses or in superscript, depending upon the journal's editorial style. The following are three examples of reference citations in the text, using the citation order system:

- The exact etiology of congenital skeletal limb deficiencies is unknown (1).
- Several studies (4–6) have examined the impact of technology on the care of the elderly.
- The health professional's viewpoint of disability can differ from that of the parent of a child who is handicapped (4, 10, 15).

In the first example, only one reference is being cited and it is the first to appear in the text. In the second example, the writer is referring to three publications which appear in consecutive order in the text. Three references are cited in the third example, however, they do not appear in consecutive order in the text.

Alphabet-Number System

The alphabet-number system is similar to the citation order system in that each work cited in the text, is assigned a number. However, it differs from the citation order system in that the assigned number corresponds to the alphabetical listing of the reference at the end of the paper; in the reference list, the works are listed in alphabetical order and are numbered serially. The number appropriate to each reference is used to cite the work in the text; at the proper point in the text, the number is typed in superscript or is placed in parentheses, depending upon the style adopted by the journal.

Although both these methods of reference citations tend to reduce the length of the text and consequently, the cost for the number of words printed, the reader must consult the reference list (at the end of the paper), to identify the works being cited. For some readers, this is considered to be a disadvantage as it cuts the flow of thought while reading the narrative text. However, from the writer's viewpoint, both these methods are relatively easy to use; regardless of the number of works or the number of authors being cited, the reference in the text is always cited in the same way (i.e., by a number).

Author-Date System

The author-date (or name and year) system, as proposed by the American Psychological Association (1983), is the one which has been adopted by many health journals. If the journal to which you are submitting your manuscript uses this method, it is strongly recommended that you consult this third edition of the *Publication Manual of the American Psychological Association,* for more complete and detailed information.

Basically, this method of citation is characterized by identifying for each publication cited, the author's surname and the year of publication. The reader can locate the cited work by consulting the alphabetical reference list at the end of the paper. Depending upon the number of works and the number of authors being cited, the reference in the text is presented differently. Let us look at some of the basic rules of this method, when citing one work by a single author; one work by two or more authors; and two or more works by different authors.

One Work by a Single Author: In the following four examples, one work by a single author is cited in the text:

- Levy (1985) estimates that the number of nurses ...
- In 1986, Moore reported a high incidence ...
- In a study on children with speech problems (Dudley, 1982), the results showed that ...
- He reported that "biofeedback was an effective means for reducing the degree of shoulder subluxation in adults with hemiplegia" (Truman, 1984, p. 15).

In the first example, only the author's surname is an integral part of the text and consequently, only the year of publication is placed in parentheses. In the second example, both the year of publication and the author's surname are part of the text and thus there is no need for any parentheses. Since the opposite is true for example 3, both the author's surname and the year of publication, separated by a comma, are placed in parentheses. In the fourth example, the source of a direct quotation is indicated; the quotation is enclosed with quotation marks, and the author's surname, the year of publication and the page number are identified.

One Work by Two or More Authors: The following four examples illustrate how to cite a publication written by two or more authors:

- According to Weiss and Dutil (1980), many therapists ...
- Only one study (Weiss & Dutil, 1980) reported that ...
- The work of Casey, Bing, Green and Walter (1988) revealed that ... [first citation]
- Casey et al. (1988) found that ... [subsequent citations]

In the first two examples, one work by two authors is being cited, but they are presented differently. In example 1, only the year of publication is not part of the text and consequently, it is placed in parentheses. In example 2, since the reference citation is not part of the text, it is placed in parentheses; note that the authors' surnames are joined by an ampersand [&], and are followed by a comma, and then by the year of publication. The third example shows that the work cited has more than two but fewer than six authors; in this case, all authors are referred to the first time the reference appears in the text. In subsequent citations, as illustrated in example 4, only the surname of the first author is identified and is followed by "et al." and the year of publication in parentheses.

Two or More Works by Different Authors: In the following example, more than two publications are cited within the same parentheses:

A number of authors (Dutil, 1970; Ferland, 1985; Hachey & Forget, 1982) investigated ...

In this example, since more than two works by different authors are being cited and are not part of the narrative, they are placed within the same parentheses, in alphabetical order by the first author's surname. Note that the citations are separated by semicolons.

These are but a few examples of how to apply, in the text, the author-date method of citation (American Psychological Association, 1983). It is important to vary (as illustrated in these examples) the presentation of the literature cited, as it makes for more interesting reading. Remember to pay close attention to the accuracy of the punctuation and spelling of the reference citation.

One advantage of this citation method is that the text quickly points out the source of the information to the reader, thereby eliminating the need to consult frequently the reference list at the end of the paper. On the other hand, this system incurs an expense for the journal, since the references to cited works constitute a large portion of the text; the more words printed, the greater the cost.

This section presented three of the methods used to cite references in the text of a journal publication. It is important to note that it is not you, the writer, who decides which citation method will be used; each journal specifies in its guidelines, the style it has adopted and consequently, your manuscript must adhere to that style.

A well-written literature review is one which is characterized by the following features:

1. It presents a synthesis and critical examination of the literature.
2. The information is logically organized and accurately reported.
3. The publications reviewed are relevant to the subject being addressed and are up-to-date.
4. There is no omission of any important works on the subject.
5. All the works reviewed are cited in conformance with the editorial style adopted by the journal to which the manuscript will be submitted.

METHODOLOGY

The methodology (or materials and methods) component of a journal publication describes the procedure(s) used to conduct the study. Because of its descriptive and somewhat technical nature, the methodology provides a detailed and systematic account of what was done and how it was done. It thereby enables the reader to understand the subsequent parts of the paper (i.e., results and discussion) and provides the basis for replication of the study by others.

A description of the methodology is always included in a research article and may also be presented in other types of papers, such as the new ideas report. Since this part of the manuscript is written after the study has been conducted, the elements which need to be addressed have already been considered and are now ready to be communicated in writing.

In most health professional journals, the elements constituting the methodology are presented and organized in the following order:

1. Subjects (e.g., number of subjects, age, sex, diagnosis).
2. Measuring instruments (e.g., questionnaire, interview, test or apparatus used).
3. Procedure (e.g., method of collecting the data).
4. Data analysis (e.g., method of analyzing the data).

Each of these elements must be clearly, methodically and fully described. Too much or too little information may result in the reader having difficulty understanding the content and/or in replicating the study.

How to Write the Methodology

To help you begin writing the methodology, it is suggested that you ask yourself the following questions:

Who?

Who were the subjects?
Who were the examiners?

What?

What criteria were used to select the subjects?
What parameters or variables were studied?
What tests or apparatus were used as measuring instruments?
What instructions were given to the subjects?
What research design was selected for the study?
What procedure was used to collect the data?
What method was used to analyze the data?

When?

When were the subjects tested or treated (e.g., frequency or duration of the sessions)?
When was the study conducted?

Where?

Where were the subjects selected from?
Where was the study conducted?

Why?

Why were these subjects selected?
Why were these measuring instruments used?
Why was this research design selected?
Why was this procedure used to collect the data?
Why was this method of analyzing the data chosen?

The answers to those questions which are applicable to your paper can be used to organize the methodology into the four sub-divisions: (a) subjects, (b) measuring instruments, (c) procedure, and (d) data analysis. Compose a narrative text which clearly describes each of these elements; if permitted by the journal, use sub-headings.

The following example takes one of these elements, "subjects," to illustrate how the text can be written:

> The 20 subjects of this study were 10 men and 10 women ranging in age from 18 to 48 years, with a mean age of 32.5 years. The sample group was selected from an acute rehabilitation center. All subjects had sustained traumatic amputation of their dominant upper limb and had an admitting diagnosis of below-elbow amputation (n = 10), above-elbow amputation (n = 5) or shoulder disarticulation amputation (n = 5). Table 1 presents a summary of demographic information about the subjects. All subjects read and signed a consent form before admission to the study.

When writing the methodology section, reference citations may be included but are usually few in number since this part of the paper describes what you did rather than what others did. However, if you used a measuring instrument or procedure which was previously published, you must cite the source of your information. Direct quotations are rarely presented in this part of the paper.

Figures and/or tables may be presented to clarify, document or amplify the text. They should be used only if essential and they should not repeat the information in the text. A figure, for example, may be used to illustrate the materials of a test or the design components of a measuring instrument. A table may be used to record subject data or to list test items and scoring criteria. As reported in the example above, the text must direct the reader to the figure or table being addressed by referring to its number.

RESULTS

The purpose of the results component of a journal publication is to summarily report the findings of the study. As Kittredge (1985) explains, the results section presents only the facts and does not explain what those facts mean. By presenting quantitative and/or qualitative data, this part of the paper serves to inform the reader as to what were the consequences or outcome of the investigation. Regardless of the type of information being disclosed, the results should represent meaningful data. This however, does not necessarily imply that negative results are to be excluded; meaningful results refer to relevant findings which either positively or negatively affect the variables studied.

A disclosure of the results is always included in a research article and may also be presented in other types of papers (e.g., case or clinical report), even though a heading is not always used to label this section. This part of the manuscript is written after the data have been objectively and critically examined. If statistics were used, it is strongly recommended that authors, who are not proficient in analyzing and reporting statistical data, should consult with a biostatistician.

A well-written results section is characterized by the following features:

1. Only the findings of the study are disclosed; any description of the methodology or interpretation of the data is reserved for the methodology and discussion sections respectively.

2. The results reported are meaningful; findings which are not relevant to the outcome of the study, are excluded.

3. The tables and figures used to record and summarize the results provide information which is supplemental and essential to the narrative text; the number of tables and illustrations is appropriate and repetitive data are not included.

4. The narrative text cites the number of the table or figure being reported and guides the reader's attention to what is being examined; a

table or figure should not be presented without it being mentioned in the text.

5. The textual matter is presented objectively, briefly, succinctly and accurately; the use of verbose or repetitive text is avoided.

How to Write the Results

Before beginning to write the results component, it is suggested that you first decide which results of the study will be included in your manuscript, and which will be excluded. That is, you must discriminate between those findings which are meaningful, would be of interest and value to the readers, and therefore should be reported and those results which are not relevant, would not be of interest and value to the readers, and consequently, should not be presented. Some novice health professional writers do not make this distinction because they tend to think that all the data analyzed must be reported; as a result, this part of the paper is often poorly written and does not meet the criteria for journal publication. The converse of this fault may also be true; too little or a lack of data may not provide sufficient information to justify the conclusion of the study and consequently, the results section requires rewriting.

Once you have identified which results you intend to disclose, you need to determine how this information can best be reported. Will the findings be presented only in narrative form, or will certain results be revealed in the form of tables and/or figures which supplement the text? If you have selected the latter approach, you should be able to justify the value and need for each table or figure used. Some health professional writers prefer to determine the content of the tables and figures, as well as the order in which they will be presented, before transcribing the data into textual matter.

TABLES AND FIGURES

In a journal publication, tables and figures are used to present information which supplements the narrative text. A table is a systematic arrangement of either numerical data or textual matter and hence, can be of a quantitative or qualitative nature. A figure, on the other hand, is a graphic representation of narrative text, primarily in the form of photographs, graphs, line drawings, or charts.

The purpose of tables and figures is to add essential information to the narrative text. They are not used to repeat or duplicate the textual matter, but rather to clarify, simplify, amplify or record information which is supplemental and essential to the text. The reader should be able to understand the table or figure, without having to read the text; they should be self-explanatory. The text however, should guide the reader's attention to what is to be examined in the table or figure. When submitted, each table and figure is presented on a separate page, and when published, each is placed as close to the text as possible.

Every table and figure must have a number and a title. Tables and figures are numbered consecutively in the order in which they first appear in the text. The title follows this number, and clearly and briefly describes the content of the table or figure. Depending upon the journal's style, the number and title appear either on top of or below the body of the table or figure.

The body (or contents) of a table presents the numerical data or textual matter, in a clear, logical and systematic arrangement; an overwhelming amount of data or a complicated composition should be avoided. The body of a figure refers to the graphic illustration in the form of a photograph, graph, line drawing or chart. Below the body of a table or figure, footnotes, legends or captions can be presented to explain or provide additional information. These notes can also be used to acknowledge the copyright source of any reproduced material. Both tables and figures are assessed for their size and proportion, clarity, accuracy, consistency, readability and simplicity.

How to Prepare Tables and Figures

Tables and figures are complicated and expensive to publish, and for this reason, you should be able to justify their need and value for the reader. To help you determine whether or not to include a table or figure in your manuscript, ask yourself the following questions:

What information do you want to present in the form of a table or figure?
Is this information of a quantitative or qualitative nature?
Why do you feel that this information should be presented in tabular or graphic form, rather than as textual matter?
What is the purpose of the table or figure?
What type of table or figure best suits this purpose?
What is the proportionate value of each table or figure?

By answering these questions, you will have justified the need for and the value of your tables and figures. You can now proceed to preparing them in conformance with the guidelines of the journal to which the manuscript will be submitted. If you do not have the skill or expertise for producing a quality figure, consult with someone who has, for example, a professional artist or medical photographer. You may also want to consider the amazing virtuosity of the computer-as-artist; today's ever-expanding world of computers can provide you with the means of producing computer-generated tables and figures of outstanding quality.

If the table or figure you are presenting is not your own, you are responsible for obtaining permission to use it in your paper; written permission from the copyright source must be obtained to reproduce or adapt, all or part of a table or figure, which was taken from a previously published source. In addition, you must identify the copyright source and acknowledge that permission to reprint the material was granted.

DISCUSSION

The discussion component of a journal publication discloses the author's evaluation and interpretation of that which was examined in the paper. By showing relationships among those facts reported in other parts of the paper, particularly the results section, the author discusses the problem or subject being investigated. The conclusion can be an integral part of the discussion, or it can be presented as a separate component, under the heading "conclusion."

All research articles must include a discussion of the results reported in the preceding part of the paper. Even though a journal publication may not include a results component (as in the case of a review or theoretical article), it almost always presents a discussion of the issues under examination. Consequently, the way in which the discussion is written will vary slightly, depending upon the type of publication. For the most part however, this section focuses on how the discussion is presented in a research article.

The discussion part of a journal publication has the distinct characteristic of bringing into relation the facts or observations reported in the (a) literature review, (b) methodology, and (c) results components of the paper:

a. Relation between the literature review and the discussion; the results of the study are critically examined by comparing them to the findings reported in the literature review.
b. Relation between the methodology and the discussion; the results are explained and interpreted by associating them with the procedure(s) described in the methodology section.
c. Relation between the results and the discussion; the findings reported in the results section are evaluated and interpreted by the author.

How to Write the Discussion

Of all the components of a journal publication, you will probably find that the discussion is one of the most difficult to write. It requires that you possess not only good writing skills, but also a particular capacity to reason, to debate, to synthesize and to formulate a sound opinion. In the preceding parts of your paper, your personal viewpoint was not expressed. That is, in the literature review, you surveyed what other authors reported; in the methodology, you described the procedure(s) used to conduct your study; and in the results section, you presented the data you analyzed. Now, in the discussion part of the paper, you can and should express your own comments, opinions or arguments regarding the meaning of your results. Although your point of view might differ from that of some of the readers, you are entitled to an opinion based on the evidence reported.

It is best to write the discussion after you have written the preceding parts of the manuscript. Before beginning to write the discussion, it might be helpful for you to address the following questions:

What general principles or relations can be inferred from your results?

How are the results of your study in agreement or disagreement with the findings reported in your literature review?

How does your interpretation of the results differ from or is similar to those works reviewed in your literature review?

What are the methodological limitations of your study?

What are the theoretical or clinical implications of your findings?

What recommendations do you suggest for future studies?

What is the underlying significance of the results?

The last three questions pertain more directly to the conclusion(s) which can be drawn and consequently, they can be addressed either when writing the discussion or the conclusion component of your paper.

Your answers to these questions should help you to begin writing the discussion. Organize the information into a logical order; usually, the general organization of the discussion component is similar to that used to present the results. For example, if the results section presented descriptive statistics (e.g., means or standard deviations) before inferential statistics (e.g., t tests, F tests, chi-square), then the data is generally discussed in the same order.

CONCLUSION

The purpose of the conclusion is to bring the paper to an end, by signifying the final outcome or judgment drawn from the work. Based on the reported evidence, the conclusion is derived through logical deduction. In other words, on the basis of the established findings and through the process of scientific reasoning, the author reaches a final decision or opinion as to the significance of the work.

Most journal publications have a conclusion and if necessary, more than one can be presented. The conclusion is usually presented as a separate component (with its own heading), but can also be an integral part of the discussion section. If no definite conclusion can be drawn, the author may prefer to end the paper with a summary rather than a conclusion; this is generally acceptable, provided that the summary ends the paper by presenting a comprehensive synopsis of the paper's content.

How to Write the Conclusion

The conclusion is one of the last components of a journal publication to be read as well as written. Before composing the text for the conclusion, ask yourself three important questions:

1. What are the theoretical or clinical implications of the study?
2. What is your final opinion, decision or recommendation on the subject?
3. What is the underlying significance of your work?

Your answers to these questions will help you begin composing the text for the conclusion. In writing (and rewriting) this component, it is important that you do not try to impress the reader by extrapolating the findings or the significance of your work. Many novice health professional writers tend to project, expand, or predict the meaning of their data or findings and write very lengthy conclusions; this is not recommended in writing a journal publication. Your conclusion should be based on reported evidence and scientific reasoning, and should be written as clearly and as briefly as possible.

ACKNOWLEDGMENTS

The acknowledgments is that component of a journal publication in which the author formally and favorably recognizes the participation and assistance of any persons and/or agencies who significantly contributed to the work in question. It is simply an expression of thanks or gratitude and its inclusion in the paper is left to the discretion of the author.

In a journal publication, the type of assistance which is usually acknowledged, includes the following:

1. Financial support in the form of grants or fellowships.
2. Participation of subjects, patients, technicians and/or clinicians.
3. Collaboration of hospitals, centers, institutions or schools.
4. Preparation of illustrations.
5. Compilation and analysis of data.

It is not necessary to recognize the assistance of those persons whose regular duties required them to participate in the work (e.g., secretaries).

The placement of the acknowledgments in the publication will vary. In some journals, it is presented after the main body of the text and before the reference list, while in others, the acknowledgments follows the authors' names and affiliations, and precedes the abstract.

How to Write the Acknowledgments

This component of a journal publication is usually written in one or two paragraphs, under the heading "acknowledgments." In expressing your thanks, be courteous, simple and brief. The following is an example which illustrates how the acknowledgments can be written:

This study was supported by a research grant from the Cerebral Palsy Association of America. The authors wish to thank the children and staff of the Shriner's Hospital, for their participation; Tom Post, for assistance in analyzing the data and Sheila Smith, for the preparation of the illustrations.

REFERENCES

In a journal publication, all references cited in the text are listed at the end of the paper, under the heading "references." The purpose of this part of the paper is to provide the reader with sufficient bibliographic information for identifying and retrieving each of the references. Only those works which were referred to in the text are presented; any references which were not cited in the text but which were consulted or are recommended for further reading, should not be included in the reference list, but rather should be presented in a bibliography.

Each journal specifies in its guidelines for authors, the style it has adopted for the presentation of references, both in the text and in the reference list. Regardless of which style is required, it is important that the way in which the references are listed at the end of the paper, is consistent and corresponds with the method used to cite the references in the text.

Types of Reference Styles

Although there are many reference styles, most health professional journals use one of three methods for listing the references at the end of the paper: (a) the citation order system, (b) the alphabet-number system, and (c) the American Psychological Association (APA) reference style.

a. The citation order system: This reference style presents a numerical listing of the references, according to the order in which they first appear in the text. In other words, beginning with the number "1," each work in the reference list is assigned a number which corresponds to the order in which the work is first mentioned in the text.

b. The alphabet-number system: The principle characteristic of the alphabet-number system is that the references are listed alphabetically by the first author's surname, and are numbered serially, with one reference per number. The number appropriate to each reference is used to cite the work in the text.

c. The APA reference style: As proposed by the American Psychological Association (1983), the APA reference style is described in detail in the third edition of their publication manual. In applying this style, the references cited in the text, are listed at the end of the paper, in alphabetical order by the first author's surname. The reference list does not include personal communications, but rather only works which can be retrieved. The types of works which are usually referenced include periodicals, books, technical and research reports, proceedings of meetings and symposiums, master's theses, doctoral dissertations, as well as unpublished manuscripts and publications of limited circulation.

When comparing these three reference styles, certain similarities and differences regarding the order in which the references are listed, should be noted.

The alphabet-number system is similar to the APA reference style in that both styles list the references in alphabetical order. However, unlike the APA style, the alphabet-number system assigns a number to each of the works presented in the reference list and uses this number (rather than the author's surname and the year of the publication), to cite the work in the text.

Although both the alphabet-number system and the citation order system use numbers to identify the references, the methods used to assign these numbers differ. With the alphabet-number system, the number assigned to the reference corresponds to the alphabetical order in which the references are listed; with the citation order system, the number assigned to the reference, corresponds to the order in which the reference first appears in the text.

Each of these reference styles has their own rules and guidelines which usually differ in terms of the elements constituting the reference, the order in which these elements are presented, and the principles of style and punctuation which must be observed.

To illustrate the application of one reference style, let us briefly examine how the APA reference style is used to reference the two most common types of works: periodicals and books.

Reference to a Periodical

In presenting a reference to a periodical, the elements to be included in the reference and the order in which they are to appear, is as follows:

1. Author's surname and initials.
2. Year of the publication.
3. Full title of the article.
4. Full title of the journal.

5. Volume number of the journal.
6. Page numbers of that volume.

The following is an example of a journal article by a single author:

Pagonis, J. F. (1987). Successful proposal writing. *American Journal of Occupational Therapy, 41,* 147–151.

The following is an example of a journal article by two or more authors:

Manchester, J., Eastland, M., & Sugden, J. (1985). Sexuality. *Nursing, 2,* 1026–1028.

In both these examples of a reference to a periodical, it is important to note some of the APA's principles of style and punctuation:

1. The surnames and initials of all authors are given.
2. Commas are used to separate authors and to separate surnames and initials.
3. In a multiple-authored work, an ampersand (&) is used before the last author's surname.
4. The year of the publication is placed in parentheses, and is followed by a period.
5. Only the first word of the article's title (and subtitle) is capitalized.
6. The title of the article is followed by a period.
7. The journal title is typed in uppercase and lowercase letters.
8. The title and volume number of the journal are italicized.
9. Commas are placed after the journal title and volume number.
10. Inclusive page numbers of the volume are given and a period ends the reference.

Reference to a Book

In presenting a reference to a book, the elements constituting the reference and the order in which they are to appear, is as follows:

1. Author's or editor's surname and initials.
2. Year of the publication.
3. Full title of the book.
4. City (or city and state) of the publisher.
5. Name of the publisher.

The following is an example of a reference to an entire book:

Isaac, S., & Michael, W. B. (1971). *Handbook in research and evaluation.* San Diego, CA: Edits Publisher.

The following is an example of a reference to a chapter in an edited book:

McDonald, E. T., & Aungst, L. F. (1970). An abbreviated test of oral stereognosis. In J. F. Bosma (Ed.), *Second symposium on oral sensation and perception* (pp. 384–390). Springfield, IL: Charles C Thomas.

As show in these two examples of a reference to a book, the principles of style and punctuation are similar to those used in a reference to a periodical:

1. The surnames and initials of all authors (or editors) are given.
2. Commas are used to separate authors and to separate surnames and initials.
3. The year of the publication is placed in parentheses and is followed by a period.
4. Only the first word of the book's title (and subtitle) is capitalized, and the title is italicized.
5. A period follows the title of the book and ends the reference.

Unlike a periodical reference, a book reference includes the city of the publisher and the name of the publisher; a colon separates these two elements.

How to Write the References

Writing the reference list first requires that you identify the reference style adopted by the journal to which your manuscript will be submitted. Read attentively the journal's guidelines for authors and ascertain which reference style must be used. Follow meticulously the instructions for presenting the references and prepare them in conformance to that style's rules or guidelines. In writing each reference, consider the type of work being referenced, the elements which should constitute the reference, and the principles of style and punctuation which are to be observed. List the works in the order specified by the reference style you are using.

A well-written list of references is one which is distinguished by the following three characteristics:

1. The references are presented in conformance with the style rules and guidelines established by the journal to which the manuscript will be submitted.

2. The information presented for each reference is accurate and complete.
3. All references listed have a corresponding citation in the text.

Before closing this chapter, it is important to point out one general principle common to writing all the components of a journal publication: *several drafts of each part of the paper need to be written until the manuscript is completed and ready to be submitted for review.* Rewriting is a pre-requisite for a quality paper. In rewriting each part of the paper, be sure that:

1. The writing style is characterized by logical organization and the use of precise and concise words.
2. The amount of detail conforms to the level of the intended reading audience.
3. The syntax, grammar, spelling and punctuation are correct.
4. The editorial style used conforms to that adopted by the journal to which the manuscript will be submitted.

QUESTIONS? ANSWERS

Question

The purpose of my paper is to review studies which have examined the problems health professionals encounter in patient-therapist relations. With the intention of attracting a large reading audience and of using an original title, I entitled my paper, "To be, or not to be: That is the problem." The journal reviewers, who evaluated my manuscript, considered this title to be too general. What would be a better title for my paper?

Answer

The purpose of the title of a journal publication is to identify the subject matter and to appeal to the intended reading audience. Your title does not do either and as a result, must be improved.

Although you wanted to attract a large reading audience by using an original title, the reader does not in any way know what subject is being addressed and for whom the paper is intended. To help you write a better title, consider the characteristics of the four types of titles described in this chapter. If you have difficulty generating ideas for your title, examine the titles of those articles you have reviewed and use them as a model for creating a meaningful title. A more appropriate title for your paper might be "Patient-therapist relations: A review of the literature."

Question

In their review of my manuscript, the journal reviewers found the title of my work to be too specific and too long. I do not feel that I should have to change it since I have seen titles of other journal publications which are just as long. If the reviewers want me to change my title, why did they not provide me with one which they considered to be acceptable?

Answer

From what you have said, it appears that you have two problems: one is your title, and the other is your attitude. Although there is no rule which states the minimum and maximum number of words that are to constitute a title, the reviewers recommended that your title be revised. Your response to this remark appears to be both negative and unprofessional. Regardless if other papers have titles which are just as long as yours, what is important is that the reviewers of your manuscript recommended that it be shortened. It is your responsibility, and not that of the reviewers to make the necessary revisions of your manuscript. A health professional who writes for publication must be open to criticism. If your reaction to other comments provided by the reviewers is the same as this, you will probably never see your paper in print.

Question

In the literature review of my manuscript, I presented a total of 20 direct quotations. Although I correctly and accurately cited the material from the authors' works, the journal reviewers were of the opinion that there were too many direct quotations. They also recommended that I obtain written permission from the copyright owners, to use each of these quotations. How can I resolve this problem?

Answer

Many novice health professional writers tend to use an overabundance of direct quotations in the literature review, primarily because they have difficulty paraphrasing the findings of the works reviewed. I suggest that you closely examine why you used each quotation. In general, you should use a direct quotation only because you feel it is important to quote the author, word for word, and not because it is difficult for you to use your own words to report published material. Although there is no rule as to the maximum number of quotations which can be used, it does make for better and easier reading if their number is kept to an essential minimum.

When quoting at length copyrighted material, it is your responsibility to write to the copyright owner to determine whether permission to quote is required, and if it is, a letter of permission must be secured and submitted together with your manuscript, to the journal's editor. You are also required to acknowledge in your paper that permission to quote was granted by the owner of the copyright.

Question

The purpose of my paper, "Sexual rehabilitation of adults with spinal cord injury," is to report to health professionals on the importance of sexuality counseling in the total rehabilitation of spinal cord-injured patients. In order to describe certain techniques of stimulation and positioning, I presented several explicit illustrations which supplemented the narrative text. The journal reviewers of my manuscript considered these illustrations to be unsuitable for publication. What should I do?

Answer

Each journal has its own policies and standards regarding the material which is considered to be suitable for publication. Although I have not read your manuscript, it appears that your illustrations did not meet the standards of the journal to which you submitted your work; perhaps the illustrations were too explicit or somewhat risqué.

Rather than submit your manuscript to another journal and risk receiving the same criticism, I would suggest that you objectively evaluate the worth and need for your illustrations, in light of the reviewers' comments. Ask yourself if these illustrations would be of greater value to patients with spinal cord injury, rather than to the health professionals reading your paper. If this is the case, perhaps your illustrations would be more appropriate in a sex education booklet designed for these patients.

It is important to bear in mind that when graphically illustrating information of a delicate nature (e.g., sexual, racial, religious), the author of a journal publication does not have as much freedom as the author of a book; you should accept this fact and conform to the policies and standards of the journal so that your paper will be acceptable for publication.

Question

The journal to which I submitted my manuscript, uses the APA reference style. I do not understand why the journal reviewers remarked that my reference list was not presented in conformance with the rules and guidelines of this style. For example, what is wrong with the way in which I presented the following reference?

D. Heming. The Titanic Triumvirate: Teams, Teamwork and Team-building. *CJOT,* 55, 15–20, 1988.

Answer

In applying the APA reference style to this reference, five corrections need to be made:

1. The author's initial should follow the surname.
2. Only the first word of the article's title and subtitle must be capitalized.
3. The name of the journal should be given in full.
4. The volume number of the journal should be italicized.
5. The year of the publication should be placed in parentheses and should follow the author's surname and initials.

The correct way in which to write this reference would be:

Heming, D. (1988). The titanic triumvirate: Teams, teamwork and teambuilding. *Canadian Journal of Occupational Therapy, 55,* 15–20.

REFERENCES AND SUGGESTED READINGS

References

American Psychological Association. (1983). *Publication manual of the American Psychological Association* (3rd ed.). Washington, DC: Author.

Cook, H. L., Beery, M., Sauter, S. V. H., & DeVellis, R. F. (1987). Continuing education for health professionals. *American Journal of Occupational Therapy, 41,* 652–657.

Cox, R. C., & West, W. L. (1982). *Fundamentals of research for health professionals.* Laurel, MD: RAMSCO.

Day, R. A. (1979). *How to write and publish a scientific paper.* Philadelphia, PA: ISI Press.

Heming, D. (1988). The titanic triumvirate: Teams, teamwork and teambuilding. *Canadian Journal of Occupational Therapy, 55,* 15–20.

Isaac, S., & Michael, W. B. (1971). *Handbook in research and evaluation.* San Diego, CA: Edits Publisher.

Kittredge, P. (1985). Writing a research paper: Basic organization and a checklist. *Respiratory Care, 30,* 1057–1061.

Manchester, J., Eastland, M., & Sugden, J. (1985). Sexuality. *Nursing, 2,* 1026–1028.

McDonald, E. T., & Aungst, L. F. (1970). An abbreviated test of oral stereognosis. In J. F. Bosma (Ed.), *Second symposium on oral sensation and perception* (pp. 384–390). Springfield, IL: Charles C Thomas.

Pagonis, J. F. (1987). Successful proposal writing. *American Journal of Occupational Therapy, 41,* 147–151.

Seeger, M. W., & Furst, D. E. (1987). Effects of splinting in the treatment of hand contractures in progressive systemic sclerosis. *American Journal of Occupational Therapy, 41,* 118–121.

Tomlinson, A., & Williams, A. (1985). Communication skills in nursing: A practical account. *Nursing, 2,* 1121–1123.

Weaver, S. A., Lange, L. R., & Vogts, V. M. (1988). Comparison of myoelectric and conventional prostheses for adolescent amputees. *American Journal of Occupational Therapy, 42,* 87–91.

Wilgosh, L. R., & Skaret, D. (1987). Employer attitudes toward hiring individuals with disabilities: A review of the recent literature. *Canadian Journal of Rehabilitation, 1,* 89–98.

Suggested Readings

American Psychological Association. (1983). *Publication manual of the American Psychological Association* (3rd ed.). Washington, DC: Author.

Beatty, W. K. (1979). Searching the literature and computerized services in medicine: Guides and methods for the clinician. *Annals of Internal Medicine, 91,* 326–332.

Binger, J. L., & Jensen, L. M. (1980). *Lippincott's guide to nursing literature: A handbook for students, writers, and researchers.* Philadelphia, PA: J. B. Lippincott.

Cremmins, E. T. (1982). *The art of abstracting.* Philadelphia, PA: ISI Press.

Day, R. A. (1979). *How to write and publish a scientific paper.* Philadelphia, PA: ISI Press.

Fuller, E. O. (1984). Preparing an abstract of a nursing study. *Rehabilitation Nursing, 9,* 32–33.

Hill, M., & Cochran, W. (1977). *Into print: A practical guide to writing, illustrating, and publishing.* Los Altos, CA: William Kaufman.

Huth, E. J. (1982). *How to write and publish papers in the medical sciences.* Philadelphia, PA: ISI Press.

MacGregor, A. J. (1979). *Graphics simplified: How to plan and prepare effective charts, graphs, illustrations, and other visual aids.* Toronto: University of Toronto Press.

Morton, L. T. (1979). *How to use a medical library* (6th ed.). London: William Heinemann Medical Books.

Reynolds, L., & Simmonds, D. (1981). *Presentation of data in science.* Boston: Martinus Nijhoff Publishers.

Roper, F. W., & Boorkman, J. A. (1984). *Introduction to reference sources in the health sciences* (2nd ed.). Chicago: Medical Library Association.

Warner, S. D., & Schweer, K. D. (1982). *Author's guide to journals in nursing and related fields.* New York: Haworth Press.

Chapter III

TYPES OF JOURNAL PUBLICATIONS

Either write things worth reading or do things worth writing.
Benjamin Franklin

Health professional journals differ with respect to what kinds of papers they publish. Depending upon the journal's philosophy, objectives and priorities, the types of publications which are featured will vary. These journals also differ with regards to the criteria they use to review manuscripts; each journal has its own criteria for evaluating a manuscript's suitability for publication. Some journals use a comprehensive set of general criteria for evaluating all types of journal manuscripts; some apply specific criteria for different types of manuscripts; while others identify the parts of the manuscript which are to be evaluated and the reviewers appraise each of these components using their own criteria. Because the review criteria are not the same for all health professional journals, and because there are differences in reviewers' levels of expertise and experience, it is possible for a manuscript to be accepted by one journal even though it was rejected by another.

Taking into consideration these important factors, this chapter focuses on ten types of journal publications which the health professional would most likely be interested in learning how to write (see Table IV). These ten types of papers have been grouped into three main categories: (a) feature articles, (b) brief reports, and (c) views and reviews. The primary goal and principle characteristics of each type of journal publication are described. As a guideline to learning how to prepare and write the various types of manuscripts, examples of published articles are examined, and the review criteria and evaluation forms used by some journals are presented. Additional manuscript review forms are presented in Appendix B: *American Journal of Occupational Therapy* (Appendix B.1); *Archives of Physical Medicine and Rehabilitation* (Appendix B.2); *Canadian Journal of Occupational Therapy* (Appendix B.3); *Journal of Allied Health* (Appendix

59

B.4); *Journal of Nursing Administration and Nurse Educator* (Appendix B.5); and, *Rehabilitation Nursing* (Appendix B.6).

TABLE IV
TYPES OF JOURNAL PUBLICATIONS IN THE HEALTH FIELD

Feature Articles
Descriptive article
review article
theoretical article
description of a new approach, program or service
Research article
Brief Reports
New ideas report
Case report
Clinical report
Opinion report
Views and Reviews
Letter to the editor
Book review

It is important to bear in mind that the criteria used to evaluate your manuscript depends on the journal to whom you submit your work, and therefore, the review criteria presented in this chapter should be considered only as an instructional tool for learning how to write a journal manuscript that will qualify for publication.

FEATURE ARTICLES

Feature articles constitute the first category of journal publications. A feature (or lead) article in a health professional journal, can be defined as a full-length (12–18 pages) paper that presents an original work in the field of health science. This type of paper provides new and important theoretical, clinical, or basic information which contributes to the advancement of knowledge and practice of one or more health disciplines.

The length of a feature article will vary, however it usually does not exceed 20 double-spaced typewritten pages (5,000–6,000 words), including references, tables and figures. Manuscripts of this kind always begin with an abstract and introduction. They end with a conclusion (or summary) and a list of references; at the discretion of the author, acknowledgments may or may not be included. The component parts constituting the main body of text varies, depending upon the type of feature article selected.

The category of feature articles can be divided into two main groups: descriptive and research articles.

Descriptive Articles

Descriptive articles include reviews of literature, presentations of theory, and descriptions of a new approach, program or service. Although these three types of papers differ in their goals and content, they have been grouped together mainly because of the following characteristics: (a) They are descriptive in nature, (b) they do not present numerical data or statistical analyses, and (c) they are similar in their format and as such, the same criteria are often used for review purposes.

Review Article

A review article is basically an exhaustive review of the literature, whereby the author presents a succinct and coherent analysis of the current state of knowledge on a particular subject. This type of paper provides a critical review of the literature, in a new and different perspective. It can address basic, clinical or professional issues, as well as examine a subject from an historical viewpoint.

Writing a good review article can be difficult and time-consuming. Not all health professionals can write this type of paper because it requires certain writing skills; the ability to assimilate, evaluate, organize and synthesize a large number of published works and to combine diverse concepts, findings or observations into a coherent whole. The following is an example of a review article:

Ince, L. P., Leon, M. S., & Christidis, D. (1985). EMG biofeedback for improvement of upper extremity function: A critical review of the literature. *Physiotherapy Canada, 37,* 12–17.

This review article critically examines the clinical applications of electromyographic (EMG) biofeedback for the improvement of upper extremity function, with persons who are physically disabled. The paper is written primarily for physical therapists who use EMG biofeedback and who wish to know the present state of knowledge on this subject.

In the introduction, the authors explain that in order to determine the effectiveness of this treatment modality, for this particular group of clients, a review of the works that have been done to date is necessary. The content of the paper is divided into four main therapeutic topics: the reduction of muscle spasticity and the increase of muscle activity; the increase of range of motion; the elimination of undesirable movements; and the relation between biofeedback and physical therapy. The authors provide a synthesis of 37 works and critically review them in terms of their methodology and results. The discussion focuses on which aspects of EMG biofeedback need further investigation. The conclusion drawn from this critical review emphasizes the need for further study of this treatment modality. This paper is an important contribution to the field of physical therapy, as well as to other health professions interested in the clinical application of EMG biofeedback.

Theoretical Article

A theoretical article serves to describe and discuss theoretical issues critically. It provides a theoretical framework for understanding a particular subject. The health professional writing this type of paper must not only have a clear understanding of the theoretical principles, concepts and implications being examined, but must also be proficient in organizing and communicating this information. The following is an example of a theoretical article:

Krebs, D. E. (1987). Measurement theory. *Physical Therapy, 67,* 1834–1839.

Although this theoretical article was published in *Physical Therapy,* the audience of readers is not limited to physical therapists; all health professionals use assessment instruments and therefore, the subject of this paper, measurement theory, should be of interest to a wide audience of readers.

In the introduction, the author states that the purpose of this article is to lay the conceptual foundation of concrete measurement applications. The content is organized under the following subheadings: data classification; operationalization; logical and statistical considerations; performance stability; units and dimensions of measurement; units of analysis; and measurement meaningfulness. Twenty-four works are cited in the text, thereby providing supportive research on the subject. The importance of valid and reliable measurements is signified in the summary at the end of the paper. At the time this article was written, the author was Associate Research Scientist at New York University Post-

Graduate Medical School; his expertise in the theory and clinical application of measurement is clearly reflected in this well-written and valuable article.

Description of a New Approach, Program or Service

A description of a new approach, program or service is the type of article which can be written by health practitioners with clinical experience and expertise. It provides the reader with practical information regarding a new assessment or treatment approach, an innovative program or a different health care service. An example of this type of descriptive article appears below:

> Calder, D. A. (1985). Development of an information system for a physiotherapy department. *Physiotherapy Canada, 37*, 25–30.

This article describes the development of an information system for use by physiotherapy department directors in management planning and control. The introduction provides background information on the subject and states the purpose of the paper. Two important aspects of information systems are addressed in the content: management of information processing functions and effective use of information systems in physiotherapy departments. In addition, the author describes five steps involved in developing an information system: system analysis, selection of design approach, system design, implementation and maintenance. The conclusion stresses the importance of collecting data in a systematic, formally planned way. This article provides physiotherapy directors with practical and valuable information for implementing such a system in their department.

Criteria for Acceptable Descriptive Articles

To illustrate one journal's criteria for acceptable manuscripts of this type, the review form of *Physical Therapy* is presented in Table V. As shown, the criteria are arranged according to the components which constitute a descriptive article: abstract, introduction, content, discussion and conclusion. The descriptive article does not include a methodology and results section, but rather presents the content as an integrated whole, in the main body of text. It is in the content part of the paper that the author reviews the literature, or presents a theory or describes an approach, program or service. Although this journal identifies the discussion as being a distinct component of a descriptive article, it is often acceptable for the discussion to be an integrated part of the content, and as such, is not always identified with a heading.

The specific criteria listed here are used together with the general criteria outlined in Table I (see "General Criteria for Acceptable Journal Manuscripts" in Chap. I). Thus, all manuscripts of this type, which are submitted to *Physical Therapy,* are reviewed in terms of both general and specific criteria.

Research Articles

Research is the means by which health professions can validate the therapeutic effectiveness of their practice and establish a scientific body of knowledge as a foundation. In order to substantiate a health profession's scientific credibility, research must be conducted, disseminated and published. The purpose of a research article is to report original findings which are scientifically valid and clinically meaningful. Regardless of the nature of the research study, this type of article must adhere to the scientific method, in terms of its content and writing style. Health professionals with research expertise and competence are the most qualified to write a research article.

An examination of the number of research articles which are published by a journal is one method of measuring the research activity within a profession (Holliday, 1981). In the field of occupational therapy, for example, there has been a recent trend toward more research-based literature. In an analysis of publication trends in the *American Journal of Occupational Therapy* (AJOT) during 1970–1980, Ottenbacher and Short (1982) found that there was a significant change in the type of articles published before and after 1978; specifically, there was an increase in data-based articles labeled as quasi-experimental, while the number of articles labeled as descriptive decreased during the same period. In another study, 1,746 articles published from 1970 to 1982 inclusive, were analyzed from the AJOT, the *British Occupational Therapy Journal* (BOTJ), and the *Australian Occupational Therapy Journal* (AOTJ) (Ziviani, Behan & Rodger, 1984). With regards to article format, the results indicated that research literature had increased in both AOTJ (from 6.1% to 20.0%) and BOTJ (from 8.0% to 11.4%), while that of AJOT had remained consistent at approximately 32%. The results of these two studies reveal the development of one profession's advancement toward a research-based practice through its journal publications.

TABLE V
CRITERIA FOR ACCEPTABLE DESCRIPTIVE ARTICLES:
PHYSICAL THERAPY

FOR ALL LEAD ARTICLES   Author:
(EXCEPT RESEARCH)
Reviewer #   Title:

Description of an approach or process, review of literature, or presentation of theory.	*Not ck'd*	*Not appl.*	*Yes*	*No*	*Explanations/ Comments*
ABSTRACT					
Includes the following:					
Purpose					
Summary of key points presented					
Statement of conclusions or recommendations					
Clinical relevance (if appropriate)					
Briefly presented in 150 words or less					
Accurately conveys content					
INTRODUCTION					
Purpose is stated					
Clearly					
Early in text					
Includes scope (or limitations) of article					
Supportive rationale provided is					
Relevant					
Adequate					
Assumptions appear valid					
CONTENT					
Detail provided is					
Adequate					
Relevant					
Appropriate for purpose					
DISCUSSION					
Follows logical sequence as in organization of content					
Relevant to topic					
Includes key points related to purpose					

TABLE V (continued)

Description of an approach or process, review of literature, or presentation of theory.	Not ck'd	Not appl.	Yes	No	Explanations/ Comments
DISCUSSION (continued)					
Accurately interprets issues presented					
Relates findings to work done by others					
Discusses professional implications for use of information					
Discusses clinical relevance (if appropriate)					
Makes recommendations for further work (if appropriate)					
CONCLUSION					
Stated briefly					
Summarizes key findings and implications of findings					

Reprinted from Physical Therapy Criteria Packet Review Forms, with the permission of the American Physical Therapy Association.

The component parts constituting a research article include the following: abstract, introduction, methodology, results, discussion, and conclusion. To illustrate how this type of manuscript should be prepared, the following example of a well-written research article is presented:

> Urey, J. R., & Henggeler, S. W. (1987). Marital adjustment following spinal cord injury. *Archives of Physical Medicine and Rehabilitation, 68,* 69–74.

The purpose of this research study was two-fold: first, to examine marital characteristics of couples who are coping successfully with spinal cord injury (SCI) versus those who are not, and second, to determine the relationship of positive marital adjustment in SCI couples as compared with successful adjustment among able-bodied couples.

The content and the writing style of this article clearly reflect the scientific method inherent in research. The introduction presents the nature and scope of the problem, reviews the pertinent literature and states the purpose of the study. The method section describes the subjects, the research design, the procedure, the measurement instruments and the statistical data analysis; it provides a clear and systematic account of what was done and how it was done. The results reveal what was found and for this purpose, they are organized into two parts. The first part presents the results obtained from three assessment instruments: the Marital Activities Inventory, the Sexual Interaction Inventory and the Areas of Change Questionnaire. The second part reports the observation measures of marital communication. Four tables are included for the purpose of recording and summarizing the quantitative data; the tables provide information that is supplemental and essential to the text. In their discussion, the authors evaluate and interpret the results in relation to the findings reported in other published works. The clinical implications and significance of the study are clearly stated at the end of the discussion. In the reference list, thirty-four references are presented in accordance to the reference style adopted by *Archives of Physical Medicine and Rehabilitation*. This research article provides new and important clinical information to health professionals who treat individuals with spinal cord injuries.

Criteria for Acceptable Research Articles

As adopted by *Physical Therapy*, the specific criteria for acceptable research articles are listed on the review form presented in Table VI. The criteria are organized according to the components which constitute this type of manuscript. In addition to this list of specific criteria, the journal reviewers for *Physical Therapy* also evaluate this type of manuscript in terms of general criteria (see "General Criteria for Acceptable Journal Manuscripts" in Chap. I).

BRIEF REPORTS

The second category of journal publications is entitled "brief reports." This type of paper can best be defined by its length; it is a short manuscript (3–6 pages). Despite its length however, a journal publication of this kind is a valuable forum for sharing new and important information. Depending upon the journal's specifications, an abstract may or may not be required. This type of publication however, always begins with an introduction and ends with a short list of references. The component parts constituting the main body of text varies, depending upon the type of brief report selected.

The category of brief reports can be divided into four types of journal

TABLE VI
CRITERIA FOR ACCEPTABLE RESEARCH ARTICLES:
PHYSICAL THERAPY

FOR A REPORT ON RESEARCH					
Author:					
Reviewer #					
Title:					

	Not ck'd	Not appl.	Yes	No	Explanations/ Comments
ABSTRACT					
Includes:					
Purpose					
Method					
Subject					
Design (approach to solve problem)					
Procedures/conditions/instrumentation (steps)					
Results					
Conclusion					
Clinical relevance					
Briefly presented in 150 words or less					
Accurately conveys content					
Order of presentation follows text					
INTRODUCTION					
Problem or question clearly defined					
Supportive rationale for importance of problem:					
Relevant					
Appropriate in quantity					
Purpose of study:					
Stated clearly in text					
Consistent with text					
Type of study clarified or implied (experimental, correlational, descriptive, other)					

TABLE VI (continued)

	Not ck'd	Not appl.	Yes	No	Explanations/ Comments
INTRODUCTION (continued)					
If experimental or correlational, it must include one of the following to assure appropriate analysis of data and statement of findings:					
A statement of the null hypotheses or A statement of the expected results (research hypothesis)					
If descriptive study, it must include the following:					
Need for collecting data/reporting findings (may be included in importance of problem)					
Only data included that is pertinent to problem, purpose, and type of study					
Appropriate subheadings provided, as needed, for material such as review of literature					
METHOD					
Contains appropriate subheadings about data presented below					
Subjects adequately described:					
Number					
Characteristics					
Method of selection/assignment					
Design of study appropriate for					
Problem or question					
Purpose of study					
Type of study					
Testing expectations or null hypothesis					
Procedures/conditions/instrumentation:					
Evidence of patient protection (statement if informed consent form obtained/protocol approved)					
Appropriate for design					

TABLE VI (continued)

	Not ck'd	Not appl.	Yes	No	Explanations/ Comments
METHOD (continued)					
Described briefly but with sufficient detail or references to allow replication (greater detail if unusual)					
Operational definitions clear					
Statistical analysis of data:					
Appropriate for type of study and design					
Appropriate for testing of expectations or null hypothesis					
Appropriate for kind of data (e.g. measurement level)					
RESULTS					
Presented in order of method and data analysis sections					
Appropriate subheadings used according to method and data analysis section					
Includes only findings pertinent to problem, purpose, and type of study design and analysis of data (unless exceptional sidelights), and does not contain methods or discussion					
Data in text agree with data in figures and tables					
If data are quantitative, includes means and standard deviations or median and range					
If data analyzed for statistical significance, includes relevant critical values (such as, t, r, F, X), degrees of freedom, and obtained p values					
Data in text agree with data in figures and tables					
If data are quantitative, includes means and standard deviations or median and range					
Includes appropriate amount of written explanation of numerical data, but does not repeat all data in figures and tables					

TABLE VI (continued)

	Not ck'd	Not appl.	Yes	No	Explanations/ Comments
DISCUSSION					
Presented in logical order according to method and results sections					
Clarifies if hypothesis was accepted or rejected or if results were as expected (except for descriptive study)					
Relates to the following:					
What was done in, and obtained from, study (importance of findings)					
The problem, importance of problem, purpose of study, and either expectations and reason for them (if experimental or correlational) or need for data (if descriptive)					
Work done by others					
Summarizes clinical relevance of findings and makes practical suggestions for clinical application of results (unless research was theoretical—then states where it might lead) (A subheading, Clinical Implications, is used if possible)					
Suggests further research or additional research questions raised by study results					
CONCLUSIONS					
Stated briefly					
Summarizes only key findings and implications of study					

Reprinted from Physical Therapy Criteria Packet Review Forms, with the permission of the American Physical Therapy Association.

publications: (a) new ideas report, (b) case report, (c) clinical report, and (d) opinion report.

New Ideas Report

A new ideas report describes a new development or modification of an aid, adaptive device, prosthesis, orthosis, or technique. Some health professional journals use other titles to refer to this type of brief report, for example, "Ideas exchange" (*Canadian Journal of Occupational Therapy*), "Suggestion from the field" (*Physical Therapy*), and "Brief or new" (*American Journal of Occupational Therapy*).

Health professionals who have developed a new product or technique that would be of interest and value to their colleagues or to other health professionals, can write a new ideas report. The central focus of this type of paper is on the aid; how it was devised, designed, constructed, and clinically applied in a particular setting. A well-written new ideas report provides the reader with sufficient information to reconstruct the same device and to apply it with the type of clients for whom it was designed.

A new ideas report is generally organized as follows: introduction, literature review, description of the aid, clinical application, and discussion. An example of this type of publication is given below:

> Fairleigh, A., & Hacking, S. (1988). Post-operative metacarpophalangeal arthroplasty dynamic splint for patients with rheumatoid arthritis. *Canadian Journal of Occupational Therapy, 55,* 141–146.

This new ideas report describes the construction of a dynamic hand splint which was designed for patients with post-operative metacarpophalangeal arthroplasties. The introduction describes the nature and scope of the problem, the population for whom the splint was developed, and the need for the splint. The literature review briefly examines published works describing and comparing similar splints. This part of the paper is followed by a description of the splint; the design concept, the materials, the component parts of the splint and their function, and the method of fabrication. The clinical application of the splint in occupational therapy is then explained. In their discussion, the authors analyze the features of their splint in relation to those studies reported in the literature review. Twenty references are presented at the end of the paper, in accordance with the reference style adopted by the *Canadian Journal of Occupational Therapy.*

In this paper, the authors have also included several photographs and drawings which explain and clarify the text; these figures clearly illustrate the component parts of the splint and present different views of the splint when applied on the hand. This new ideas report provides the reader with sufficient information to reconstruct the same splint and to clinically apply it for patients with metacarpophalangeal arthroplasties.

Criteria for Acceptable New Ideas Reports

The *Canadian Journal of Occupational Therapy* (CJOT) is an official publication of the Canadian Association of Occupational Therapists. The manuscript evaluation form used by CJOT for review of this type of manuscript, is shown in Table VII. This review form identifies the parts of the manuscript which are to be evaluated; the reviewers appraise each of these components by writing their comments and recommendations on the form. In addition, a general checklist of criteria is used to complete the review of the manuscript (see Appendix B.3).

Case Report

A case report (or case study) provides a comprehensive account of an individual, with a specific clinical condition. It can either describe a person who presents an unusual problem, syndrome or disease, or it can propose an uncommon solution for treating an individual with a common problem. In both instances, the central focus of the case report is on the client; what the person's clinical condition was before and after a particular treatment intervention. By reporting facts and observations regarding the client's past and present physical, psychological and social history, this type of journal publication is aimed at providing health professionals with a new and valuable concept for treating persons with a similar clinical condition. However, because of its subjective nature and its focus on only one individual, the limitations of the case report should not be disregarded; both the author and the reader must be cautious in the generalizations and conclusions drawn from the work.

As pointed out by Vargo (1987), certain words or terms used to describe people with disabilities tend to deny these persons of the dignity and respect which is rightfully theirs. Although the term "case report" is widely and commonly used, it does have a certain negative connotation. Perhaps, a more appropriate term for this type of paper would be "client report"; instead of referring to the people we treat as "cases," we would be addressing them as individuals in a particular role.

TABLE VII
CRITERIA FOR ACCEPTABLE NEW IDEAS REPORTS:
CANADIAN JOURNAL OF OCCUPATIONAL THERAPY

MANUSCRIPT EVALUATION FORM

IDEAS EXCHANGE

REVIEWER _____ MANUSCRIPT # _____

Title

Introduction

Literature Review

Description of the Technical Device

Clinical Application of the Technical Device

Figures & Tables

Photos and Illustrations

References

Reprinted with permission from the Canadian Journal of Occupational Therapy.

A case report is generally organized into four parts: introduction, client data, treatment intervention, and discussion. The following is an example of this type of brief report:

Hunt, L. (1988). Continuity of care maximizes autonomy of the elderly. *American Journal of Occupational Therapy, 42,* 391–393.

This case report describes an occupational therapy program that solved an elderly woman's problem of self-imposed isolation in her home setting, by providing her with continuity of care and reintegration into the community. Although the problem is a common one for elderly persons who are chronically ill, the proposed treatment intervention is unique.

The introduction states the problem being examined and explains why it is worth reporting and reading. The client's data are presented by summarizing her past medical history, and the assessment findings of the neurologist, physical therapist, and occupational therapist. The occupational therapy treatment intervention for this client is described; the treatment objectives and activities of the home care program and the community-based program are explained. The duration and frequency of the therapy sessions are identified. By giving examples of how the patient improved, this part of the paper also presents the results related to the treatment intervention. In the discussion, the author explains the value of the treatment program for this particular patient, as well as for other elderly persons. Three references are listed at the end of the paper, in accordance with the reference style adopted by the *American Journal of Occupational Therapy*. Health professionals who read this case report, particularly occupational therapists, will learn a new and valuable concept for maximizing the autonomy of the elderly.

Criteria for Acceptable Case Reports

The *American Journal of Occupational Therapy* (AJOT) is an official publication of the American Occupational Therapy Association. The manuscript review form used by AJOT to evaluate case report manuscripts is presented in Table VIII. The criteria for acceptable manuscripts of this kind are presented in question form; the journal reviewers assess the manuscript by answering yes or no, to each of the questions, and if necessary, comment on their answers. The reviewers also rate the quality of various aspects of the content and rank the manuscript's suitability for publication.

Clinical Report

A clinical report (or clinical note) describes a clinical problem, intervention, program or service that is interesting, new or different. It generally focuses on an important issue in the area of practice, administration or education, and consequently, can be written by clinicians, administrators or educators. Because of its descriptive and clinical nature, it is similar to the feature article which describes a new approach, program or service. The clinical report however, differs from this type of

TABLE VIII
CRITERIA FOR ACCEPTABLE CASE REPORTS:
AMERICAN JOURNAL OF OCCUPATIONAL THERAPY

Date:

Case Report:

Please review and rate the enclosed manuscript as follows:

Content	Excellent	Very Good	Good	Fair	Poor
Purpose clearly stated in introduction					
Accurate					
Documented					
Timely					
Clear					
Organized					
Stated purpose achieved					

Criteria	Yes	No	Comments (optional)
Does this case clearly represent OT?	—	—	
Does it indicate what unique OT skills made this treatment possible? (In other words, that it could not be done by a PT, nurse, or social worker?)	—	—	
Are the OT principles that support the clinical reasoning and that explain the outcome clear?	—	—	
Are the demographic and personal data adequate to allow readers to form a picture of the patient and his or her state of health?	—	—	
Were treatment goals established through planning with the patient and family?	—	—	
Are selection of treatment modalities consistent with the patient's goals and lifestyle?	—	—	
Is the need for other appropriate rehabilitation measures indicated?	—	—	
Is it clear that adequate follow-up was carried out?	—	—	
Is the importance of function and participation in daily occupation emphasized whenever possible?	—	—	
Is the cost effectiveness of the program identified whenever appropriate?	—	—	

Disposition:

_____ Publish as is or with minor revisions.
_____ Publish after satisfactory revision and review.
_____ Borderline—doesn't fill gap in literature.
_____ Don't publish.
_____ Rank level of priority for publication (1–4). (1 is high, 4 is low).

Comments:

feature article, largely with respect to its length; a clinical report is brief (3–6 pages), and as such, there is a limited number of citations, references, tables and figures.

The clinical report is generally organized into three main parts: introduction, content (i.e., description of the problem, intervention, program or service; its application and evaluation), and conclusion (or summary). An example of this type of publication appears below:

Herring, D., King, A. I., & Connelly, M. (1987). New rehabilitation concepts in management of radical neck dissection syndrome: A clinical report. *Physical Therapy, 67,* 1095–1099.

The purpose of this clinical report is to describe a new rehabilitation concept for treating persons who have had radical neck dissection surgery due to cancer. In their introduction, the authors state the clinical problem under examination, provide some background information, and identify the purpose of the report. The content focuses on a new treatment program that was designed to provide these patients with a functional and pain-free shoulder. The program consists of passive and active range-of-motion exercises, combined with isokinetic muscle strengthening exercises. A clear and complete description of the treatment plan and its clinical application provides readers with the information needed for implementing such a program in their setting. The paper ends with a summary and a list of twelve references.

Criteria for Acceptable Clinical Reports

The manuscript review form used by *Physical Therapy* to evaluate manuscripts of this kind is presented in Table IX. In addition to this list of specific criteria, the journal reviewers for *Physical Therapy* also evaluate the manuscript in terms of general criteria (see "General Criteria for Acceptable Journal Manuscripts" in Chap. I).

Opinion Report

An opinion report presents an author's view on a timely and important issue in the area of research, practice, administration or education. By examining a particular point in question or a controversial topic, the author's opinion is presented, discussed and debated. This type of paper, thereby serves as a valuable forum for sharing views on issues which are of current interest and value to health professionals. Some health profes-

TABLE IX
CRITERIA FOR ACCEPTABLE CLINICAL REPORTS:
PHYSICAL THERAPY

FOR A CLINICAL REPORT   Author:

  Reviewer #   Title:

Describe the successful solution to a current practice problem, including patient care, education, or administrative problems.	Yes	No	Explanations/ Comments
ABSTRACT			
Includes			
Purpose			
Summary of key points presented			
Statement of conclusions or recommendations			
Clinical relevance			
Briefly presented in 150 words or less			
Accurately conveys content			
INTRODUCTION			
Background information given			
Statement made of clinical problem that necessitated the development of the process			
Purpose for reporting clearly identified			
DESCRIPTION OF A PLAN			
Organized in logical sequence			
Includes			
Statement of objectives			
Rationale for selecting components of plan			
Plan for implementing procedure			
IMPLEMENTATION OF PROCESS GIVEN BY:			
Organized in logical sequence			
Given by description of sequence of events and roles and responsibilities of persons involved in process			
EVALUATION OF EFFECT			
Organized according to process and procedures			

TABLE IX (continued)

Describe the *successful solution to a current practice problem, including patient care, education, or administrative problems.*	Yes	No	Explanations/ Comments
EVALUATION OF EFFECT (continued)			
Given by quantifiable results or description of changes resulting from application of process			
Includes strengths and weaknesses of process			
SUMMARY			
Briefly reviews key points (few sentences only)			
Makes suggestions for use of information			

Reprinted from Physical Therapy Criteria Packet Review Forms, with the permission of the American Physical Therapy Association.

sional journals use other titles to refer to this type of journal publication, for example, "The issue is" (*American Journal of Occupational Therapy*), "Commentary" (*Archives of Physical Medicine and Rehabilitation*), and "Special communication" (*Physical Therapy*).

An opinion report is generally organized into three main parts: introduction, content, and conclusion (or summary). Unlike other manuscripts submitted for review, the author's qualifications and credibility are considered as a criterion for acceptable manuscripts of this kind; the author must be recognized as being an authority on the particular subject. For this purpose, the author's identity is usually revealed to the journal reviewers. The following is an example of an opinion report:

Mueller, M. J., & Rose, S. J. (1987). Physical therapy director as professional value setter: A special communication. *Physical Therapy, 67*, 1389–1392.

The purpose of this opinion report is to discuss the physical therapy director's role as both a fiscal manager and professional value setter. The subject is an administrative issue. The introduction states the problem being examined and the purpose of the report. In the content part of the paper, the authors examine and discuss the importance for the physical therapy director to maximize the fiscal productivity and professional growth of the staff. This part of the paper is organized under the following sub-headings: administrative challenge, professional values, methods of conveying professional values, and results of the approach. The conclusion drawn from the paper emphasizes how the physical therapy director can meet this administrative challenge. At the end of the paper, fifteen references are presented in conformance to the reference style adopted by *Physical Therapy*.

When this paper was written, Mr. Mueller was Director of the Department of Physical Therapy at the Irene Walter Johnson Rehabilitation Institute, and Dr. Rose was Co-Director of the same center; both authors were recognized as being qualified to write this type of journal publication.

Criteria for Acceptable Opinion Reports

Table X presents the review form used by *Physical Therapy* to review manuscripts of this kind. The journal reviewers evaluate the manuscript using both the specific criteria listed on this form, and the general criteria outlined in Table I (see "General Criteria for Acceptable Journal Manuscripts" in Chap. I).

VIEWS AND REVIEWS

The third category of journal publications is entitled "views and reviews" and includes letters to the editor and book reviews. Unlike the feature article or the brief report, manuscripts of this kind are not reviewed by journal reviewers; the letter to the editor is reviewed by the journal's editor, and the book review is evaluated by one or two book review editors.

Letter to the Editor

A large number of health professional journals publish scholarly and intellectual letters written by their readers, in the format of a "Letter to the Editor." The purpose of this type of journal publication is to allow readers to comment on one or more articles published in the journal, or to express their opinion on issues of interest to the journal's readership. When published, the letter is often followed by a response from the original author or the editor, and thus serves as a valuable forum of dialogue.

This type of journal publication is characterized by its style; it is written in the form of a letter. The length is variable, but generally is limited to approximately 600–700 words. It is logically organized and clearly presented. The writer's opinion or comments are expressed in a

TABLE X
CRITERIA FOR ACCEPTABLE OPINION REPORTS:
PHYSICAL THERAPY

FOR A SPECIAL COMMUNICATION   Author:

Reviewer #   Title:

An opinion judged to be of interest or benefit to readers	Yes	No	Explanations/ Comments
Author Credibility			
Author is thought to have credibility in subject matter (based on author being considered by his peers to be an authority)			
Content Accuracy			
Statements seem to be true and seem to represent quoted ideas/ incidents accurately			
Documentation is provided of time, place of events, and other pertinent ideas			
Author seems to present information in an objective manner			

Reminder—

FOR *SPECIAL COMMUNICATION* papers the identity of the author is not concealed so that you can judge the credibility of the author.

Reprinted from Physical Therapy Criteria Packet Review Forms, with the permission of the American Physical Therapy Association.

thoughtful, tactful and professional manner; inflammatory, prejudicial or disparaging remarks are not acceptable for publication. Whenever possible, the writer's view is supported with references to the literature; generally, no more than five citations or references are included.

Although all health professionals can write a letter to the editor, not all letters which are submitted are published. It is the editor (and not the journal reviewers) who reviews the letter manuscript and decides whether or not it shall be published; this decision is based on the nature and quality of the letter. The criteria used for review of this type of publication are determined by the editor, and thus will vary between journals. The editor's review usually gives rise to one of three outcomes: (a) The letter is not accepted for publication, (b) the letter is accepted but requires certain editorial changes before it is published, or (c) the letter is accepted as submitted. The following is an example of this type of journal publication:

Wilson, W. F., Motley, J. V., Bradley, L. A., Blossom, D., & Tracy, T. (1988). Therapists in mental health need to become more visible. *American Journal of Occupational Therapy, 42,* 330.

In this letter to the editor, three occupational therapists and two occupational therapy assistants express their opinion regarding a previously published article:

Bonder, B. R. (1987). Occupational therapy in mental health: Crisis or opportunity? *American Journal of Occupational Therapy, 41,* 495–499.

The content of the above article prompted the writers of this letter to state their opposition to the strategy of eliminating occupational therapy in mental health. Dr. Bonder's response follows this letter and serves to clarify the issue. The original author states that although she does not support relinquishing the mental health area of practice, she believes that this elimination may occur naturally if actions are not taken to prevent it. Any misinterpretation of the author's position on the subject is thereby clarified in this professional dialogue between the readers and the author.

Book Review

Many health professional journals feature reviews of books, films, audiovisuals, journal articles and/or computer software. Although this section focuses only on the book review, many of the principles described here can also be applied when reviewing these other types of publications.

Today's market of new scholarly books in the health field is so great that it is often difficult for health professionals to decide which books are worth reading and buying. A book review that is published in a health professional journal helps readers (i.e., clinicians, researchers, educators, administrators, librarians, and students), to make this choice and thus serves as a valuable source of information.

The purpose of a book review is to summarize the major themes and overall content of the book, and to provide an objective assessment of the publication's merits and demerits. Because of these two goals, the review not only describes the book, but also offers a personal judgment of its worth.

This type of manuscript has its own length and style of organization. The length of a book review is variable and depends on the journal's specifications; some journals feature standard-length reviews (approximately 250 words) while others accept long reviews (500 to 1,000 words). A book review usually begins with the following information: the name(s) of the author(s) and/or editor(s); book title in full; volume or edition number; name and address of publisher; number of pages; year of publication; and retail price. This is followed by the review and ends with the name of the reviewer.

Most health professional journals invite their readers to become book reviewers. According to Dreher (1983), for a person to qualify as a book reviewer, three qualifications are required. The individual must have (a) the expertise on the subject matter, (b) the time available for thoroughly reading the book, and (c) the ability to be objective and honest in one's judgment. In addition to these three qualifications, a fourth can be added; the ability to write a book review that is acceptable for publication. For this purpose, many journals provide their reviewers with specific guidelines to writing this type of manuscript.

When writing a book review it is important to consider both the content and the quality of the publication. Among the questions you should ask yourself, consider the following:

Content

> For whom was the book written?
> To whom will it appeal and be of value?
> What are the major themes of the book?
> What is the nature and scope of the book?
> How is it organized?
> What is the overall value of the content?
> Does it provide new and valuable information?
> How does it compare with other books on the same or similar subject?
> What are the unique features of the book?
> Does the book meet the author's stated purpose?

Quality

> What is your opinion of the author's writing style?
> Is the writing clear, accurate and concise?
> Does the format appeal to you?
> Are the illustrations and references useful?
> Is the price affordable?
> Is the book interesting to read?
> Does it stimulate further reading?

What are the book's strengths and weaknesses?

These are but a few guiding questions to help you write a book review. For more information, it is recommended that you read and follow the book review guidelines of the journal to which your manuscript will be submitted. Reading other published book reviews can also help you learn how to write this type of journal publication.

To determine the publishable nature of the book review manuscript, an evaluation of its quality and suitability for publication is necessary. Manuscripts of this kind are usually reviewed by one or two book review editors (rather than by journal reviewers). Although the criteria used to assess book review manuscripts can vary, an acceptable book review is one that presents a summarized description of the book, and an objective and professional judgment of the publication's worth. One example of a book review appears below:

> Campbell, W. (1988). [Review of *The man who mistook his wife for a hat and other clinical tales*]. *Canadian Journal of Occupational Therapy, 55,* 213.

This book review begins by presenting the complete bibliographic information for this recent (i.e., 1987) publication. It also informs the reader that the book is available in paperback, and specifies its length (i.e., 243 pages) and price (i.e., $11.95). Following this information, the review presents an overview of the book's content and offers an objective assessment of its worth, particularly for this journal's reading audience of occupational therapists. The review is organized into four concise paragraphs.

In the first paragraph, the reviewer identifies the subject matter, indicates for whom the book was written, and provides some background information on the author. The second paragraph describes the type of book (i.e., a series of case histories) and explains how the book is organized (i.e., four parts). In the third paragraph, the reviewer offers an objective and professional assessment of the book's merits and comments on the effective and original writing style of the author. The last paragraph of this review focuses on how and why this book is worthwhile reading for occupational therapists. The book reviewer's name appears at the end of the review.

QUESTIONS? ANSWERS

Question

I would like to write a review article that critically examines a limited number of articles; five recent research studies, which have addressed the same clinical problem, would be analyzed and compared in terms of their experimental design, methods, procedures and findings. Is this acceptable, or must this type of journal article always review a large number of published works?

Answer

Some health professional journals will accept this type of review article, while others will not. For this reason, I suggest that before beginning your manuscript, you direct your question to the editor of the journal you have selected; explain the purpose of your paper and justify the need for writing and publishing this kind of review article. Depending upon the editor's answer, you will be able to decide whether or not to begin writing.

Question

My research manuscript was found to be unsuitable for journal publication; the recommendation of the peer review was that it be rejected. Among the comments and criticisms provided by the journal reviewers, the following were noted: the manuscript had no literature review section; the experimental design was unclear; the methodology section was incomplete; the statistical analysis was inappropriate; the results were presented in table form only; and the discussion did not relate the findings to previously published works. It seems that my manuscript is a perfect example of "how not to write a research article." What should I do?

Answer

My suggestions to you are as follows:

1. Read this book in its entirety and learn how to write a manuscript that has a greater potential for being published.

2. Re-evaluate whether or not you have chosen a realistic writing project.
3. Evaluate your work critically, in light of the reviewers' comments and criticisms.
4. Consider rewriting your manuscript in collaboration with an experienced writer.
5. Read other research articles and use them as a model for developing your writing skills and improving your manuscript.

Question

I developed a new and original mechanical feeder for children with cerebral palsy. I wrote a new ideas manuscript which described how the aid was designed, constructed and clinically applied. The journal reviewers of my manuscript found that in my description of the aid, there were too many drawings and photographs (i.e., ten) and too many measurements. If I do not provide all the details, the readers of my paper will not have sufficient information to reconstruct the same aid. How can I solve this problem?

Answer

Although your manuscript should provide sufficient information to enable one to reconstruct the aid, it should also be interesting to read; the reader should not be overwhelmed by the amount of detail and the number of photographs or drawings. Figures of any kind add to a manuscript's length and are costly to publish; their number should be limited to the essential minimum. It is suggested that you re-evaluate the worth and need for each of your figures. To avoid writing lengthy and complicated descriptions of how an aid was constructed, some authors summarily report the method of fabrication and invite interested readers to write to them for more detailed information. Considering this as a possible solution for improving your manuscript, I suggest that you discuss it with the journal's editor, before beginning to revise your manuscript.

Question

I am interested in writing a book review in a health professional journal. How do I apply to become a book reviewer?

Answer

The procedure is relatively simple; select the journal in which you would like to be a book reviewer, and read their guidelines for authors for information on how you must proceed. Most journals request that you write a letter to the book reviewer editor, expressing your interest in being a book reviewer. Identify your specialty area(s) and the subject matter that you are qualified to review. Indicate the number of books you would be willing to examine per year and the time period that is most convenient for you to review a publication. Include a copy of your curriculum vitae, if required. It is important to understand that once you are accepted as a book reviewer, you will be asked to submit your book review manuscript within a certain period of time; failure to do so, can result in your being dismissed as a reviewer.

REFERENCES AND SUGGESTED READINGS

References

Bonder, B. R. (1987). Occupational therapy in mental health: Crisis or opportunity? *American Journal of Occupational Therapy, 41,* 495–499.

Calder, D. A. (1985). Development of an information system for a physiotherapy department. *Physiotherapy Canada, 37,* 25–30.

Campbell, W. (1988). [Review of *The man who mistook his wife for a hat and other clinical tales*]. *Canadian Journal of Occupational Therapy, 55,* 213.

Dreher, M. C. (1983). What is a book review? *Nursing Outlook, 31,* 64.

Fairleigh, A., & Hacking, S. (1988). Post-operative metacarpophalangeal arthroplasty dynamic splint for patients with rheumatoid arthritis. *Canadian Journal of Occupational Therapy, 55,* 141–146.

Herring, D., King, A. I., & Connelly, M. (1987). New rehabilitation concepts in management of radical neck dissection syndrome: A clinical report. *Physical Therapy, 67,* 1095–1099.

Holliday, P. A. (1981). A survey of research contributions of physiotherapists. *Physiotherapy Canada, 33,* 372–376.

Hunt, L. (1988). Continuity of care maximizes autonomy of the elderly. *American Journal of Occupational Therapy, 42,* 391–393.

Ince, L. P., Leon, M. S., & Christidis, D. (1985). EMG biofeedback for improvement of upper extremity function: A critical review of the literature. *Physiotherapy Canada, 37,* 12–17.

Krebs, D. E. (1987). Measurement theory. *Physical Therapy, 67,* 1834–1839.

Mueller, M. J., & Rose, S. J. (1987). Physical therapy director as professional value setter: A special communication. *Physical Therapy, 67,* 1389–1392.

Ottenbacher, K., & Short, M. A. (1982). Publication trends in occupational therapy. *Occupational Therapy Journal of Research, 2,* 80–88.

Urey, J. R., & Henggeler, S. W. (1987). Marital adjustment following spinal cord injury. *Archives of Physical Medicine and Rehabilitation, 68,* 69–74.

Vargo, J. W. (1987). What's in a name? A note on terminology. *Canadian Journal of Rehabilitation, 1,* 75–76.

Wilson, W. F., Motley, J. V., Bradley, L. A., Blossom, D., & Tracy, T. (1988). Therapists in mental health need to become more visible. *American Journal of Occupational Therapy, 42,* 330.

Ziviani, J., Behan, S., & Rodger, S. (1984). Occupational therapy journals: The state of the art. *Australian Occupational Therapy Journal, 30,* 6–12.

Suggested Readings

American Physical Therapy Association (1982). *Advice to authors: An anthology.* Washington, DC: Author.

Cohen, H. (1988). How to read a research paper. *American Journal of Occupational Therapy, 42,* 596–600.

Currier, D. P. (1979). *Elements of research in physical therapy* (2nd ed.). Baltimore, MD: Williams & Wilkins.

DeBakey, L. (1976). *The scientific journal: Editorial policies and practices.* St. Louis, MO: Mosby.

Duffy, M. E. (1985). A research appraisal checklist for evaluating nursing research reports. *Nursing and Health Care, 6,* 539–547.

Kittredge, P. (1985). Writing a research paper: Basic organization and a checklist. *Respiratory Care, 30,* 1057–1061.

Kovacs, A. R. (1985). *The research process: Essentials of skill development.* Philadelphia, PA: F. A. Davis.

Lister, M. (1985). *Style manual for Physical Therapy: Editorial style and manuscript preparation* (5th ed.). Alexandria, VA: American Physical Therapy Association.

Maher, B. A. (1978). A reader's, writer's and reviewer's guide to assessing research reports in clinical psychology. *Journal of Consulting and Clinical Psychology, 46,* 835–838.

Mirin, S. K. (1981). *The nurses guide to writing for publication.* Wakefield, MA: Nursing Resources.

Mitcham, M. D. (1985). *Integrating research into occupational therapy: A teaching guide for academic and clinical educators.* Rockville, MD: American Occupational Therapy Foundation.

Mullins, C. J. (1977). *A guide to writing and publishing in the social and behavioral sciences.* New York: John Wiley.

Richardson, F. R. (1979). *Author's style guide to the American Journal of Occupational Therapy.* Rockville, MD: American Occupational Therapy Association.

Smith, R. V. (1984). *Graduate research: A guide for students in the sciences.* Philadelphia, PA: ISI Press.

Stein, F. (1984). *Anatomy of research in allied health* (2nd ed.). Cambridge, MA: Schenkman.

Ward, M., & Fetler, M. (1979). What guidelines should be followed in critically evaluating research reports? *Nursing Research, 28,* 120–125.

Chapter IV

BOOK WRITING

It is becoming increasingly difficult for any work which lacks the obvious earmarks of popularity to get published.

Aldous Huxley

Book publishing is a large, competitive and thriving business. The rising costs of production and merchandising however, make the process of getting published exceedingly difficult, especially for the novice writer or the unknown author. Nonetheless, today more and more health professionals are successfully achieving their goal of becoming a published book author and, as such, are contributing to the wide choice of books available in the field of health science.

To help those who aspire to writing a book-length manuscript that has potential for being published, this chapter introduces the subject of book writing. It begins with the five w's of writing a book publication. This is followed by an account of my personal trials and tribulations of book writing; suggestions on how to approach a publisher; and points to consider in a publisher-author agreement.

FIVE W'S OF WRITING A BOOK PUBLICATION
WHAT? WHO? WHY? WHERE? WHEN?

What Types of Books Can Health Professionals Write?

Generally, the types of books being written by health professionals, are either of a scientific, educational or professional nature. Unlike a journal publication, the targeted readership of a book is not limited only to health professionals; the book can be designed for a professional, student, or general public audience of readers. Depending on the subject and purpose of the book, it can address the author's peers; other health professionals; undergraduate and graduate students of health care disciplines; patients and/or their families; as well as the general public. As a result, there is a wide range of the types of books and the kinds of topics which can be written by a health professional.

Who Can Write a Book Publication?

Whether you practice as a clinician, a consultant, an educator, a researcher, or an administrator, you can write a book provided that you have the material, knowledge and expertise on the subject being addressed; the required writing skills; the qualities of a health professional writer; and the time available for writing. Thus, having an idea for a book is not sufficient for getting published; your aptitude and your attitude as a health professional writer will determine your potential in becoming a published book author.

Why Write a Book?

Health professionals who write books, do so mainly because they want to develop, disseminate and share information which would be of value to a particular audience of readers. There are of course, other reasons for writing a book (e.g., career promotion, prestige, pleasure of writing, possible financial gain), however, they are not usually the primary reason for which most health professionals write books.

Where Are Books Published?

Books written by health professionals are published throughout the world, by publishers. There are basically four publishing options to choose from: (a) commercial book publisher, (b) subsidy book publisher, (c) professional, public or private agency, and (d) self-publishing.

Although it is not easy for the unknown or novice writer to get published, a growing number of health professionals are succeeding in finding a commercial (or trade) book publisher for their work. Commercial publishers offer quality editing, design, production, advertising and sales services. Because they are responsible for all costs incurred for the publication, commercial publishers invest a considerable amount of money, expertise and time in getting the writer's work published. For those writers who are unable to find a commercial book publisher and/or who wish to pay for the publication of their work, a subsidy publisher offers an alternative means of getting published. Basically, the way in which this type of publishing program works, is that the author pays a publishing fee which is determined by the subsidy publisher; the fee varies with each manuscript, depending upon such factors as the length of the manuscript, the number of pages, the type of illustrations, and other technical factors. In return, the author receives a high percentage of the retail price of each book sold. Whether or not the author regains the publishing fee invested, depends upon how well the book sells. Having a work published by a professional, public or private agency usually does not require a financial investment by the author, and is a third alternative to getting published. There are many professional associations, and public or private organizations (e.g., hospitals, universities, government agencies), which have a publications program and are interested in publishing material written by health professionals. The fourth publishing option is self-publishing, whereby the author acts as publisher. To self-publish a book requires a considerable investment of time and money in order to produce, promote, market and distribute the book.

When Should a Health Professional Write a Book?

Just like a journal publication, there is no better time for writing a book that "write" now. The timeliness of the book is an important factor which both the writer and the publisher must consider; given the nature and scope of the book, it is more likely to interest a publisher if it differs from other competing publications, and provides readers with timely and valuable material. If you have an idea for a book-length manuscript, remember that it can take two to three years (or more) to write and publish your work. Thus, for you to write a book which has potential for being published, the timing is critical. Do not lose time talking about someday writing a book; put your pencil to the paper, or your fingers to the keyboard, and begin writing your book today.

TRIALS AND TRIBULATIONS OF BOOK WRITING

In 1981, the American Occupational Therapy Association (AOTA) published my book, "A manual for the congenital unilateral below-elbow child amputee" (Weiss-Lambrou, 1981). The AOTA gave me the opportunity of becoming a published book author and for this, I will always be grateful to them. Nonetheless, looking back now at how I approached the project of writing this manual and getting it published, I realize that I made several errors along the way. By sharing with you my trials and tribulations of book writing, I hope that you will learn from my mistakes, just as I have.

Writing the Book

After graduating from the occupational therapy program at McGill University, I practiced occupational therapy for several years at the Rehabilitation Institute of Montreal. As a therapist, I kept up-to-date with the scientific and clinical body of knowledge in occupational therapy by reading the current books and journals in the health literature. I did not however, aspire to write for publication mainly because I felt that I did not have the required writing skills. I was trained and qualified to practice occupational therapy and my writing experience was limited to patient assessment and treatment reports. Although I had certain clinical experiences and ideas which, at that time, would have been of value and interest to my colleagues, I did not communicate this knowledge in writing.

My clinical experience led me to acquire a specialized expertise in upper limb prosthetic training of both children and adults. With a desire to do research in this area, I enrolled in the master's program at Sargent College of Allied Health, Boston University. The principle objective of my research study, (Weiss, 1976) was to develop and evaluate a manual that would provide the non-expert therapist (in child prosthetics) with a working knowledge and understanding of the basic principles underlying the habilitation of the congenital, unilateral, below-elbow child amputee. Once the manual was written, ten therapists with experience in child prosthetics and ten therapists without such experience, evaluated its content and format, using a questionnaire designed for this purpose. In addition, one non-expert therapist tested the manual's first two stages of the prosthetic training program: the initial check-out evaluation of the prosthesis and the orientation stage. From the results of this study, it was concluded that there was a definite need for such a manual, and that with certain revisions, it would be a worthwhile publication.

After having successfully completed my graduate studies, I returned to Montreal to begin my career as a professor of occupational therapy at the Université de Montréal. I brought back with me the dream of one day having my book published so that it could be read by those therapists for whom it was written. Why write a book if no one reads it, I asked myself.

And so, I embarked on the journey of getting my book published. It was truly a journey since it took almost five years of unrelenting perseverance and determination until my book was published.

Getting Published

One of the first errors I committed was that in transforming part of my master's thesis into a book publication, I did not enlarge upon the subject matter, nor the size of the intended reading audience. Although the specificity of my manual's content was necessary and appropriate for a master's thesis, it was less suitable for publication in book form; the subject was too specific and the intended reading audience was too limited.

Perhaps I should have rewritten the book so that it include information on congenital and acquired amputations; the different levels of upper limb amputation (i.e., below-elbow, above-elbow, shoulder disarticulation); the degree of limb involvement (i.e., unilateral and bilateral); and the different age groups (i.e., children, adolescents and adults). If these topics were included in a book entitled for example, "Upper limb prosthetic training," the size of the reading audience would have been larger, and its potential for getting published would have been greater.

In my search for a publisher, I first considered the possibility of self-publishing my book; I would undertake all the functions of a publisher, for example, printing, advertising, and distribution. After much thought, I realized that I did not have the time, nor the money, nor the knowledge required for self-publishing and consequently, decided to find a commercial book publisher for my work.

To help me determine which publishers to approach, I looked at various books in the field of health care and identified the names of ten publishers whom I thought might be interested in my book. I made the mistake of approaching all ten publishers at the same time; I sent them each a copy of my manuscript and asked them to review it for publication purposes. This was not the best approach because it was costly in terms of both time and money. It took approximately one year until I had received an answer from all the publishers; although some promptly responded, others required several months to evaluate the publishable nature of my work. It was also an expensive approach, costing me approximately $200; each photocopy of the book was $15, plus postage and handling.

Given the nature and scope of my manuscript, the ten publishers rejected my book manuscript and gave as their reason, one of the following three explanations: (a) The subject was not compatible with their publishing program, (b) the market of potential buyers was not large enough to offset the production costs involved, or (c) the book would compete too closely with another of their own publications. Although it was never given as a reason for rejecting my manuscript, I feel that perhaps my writing credibility was questionable; I had written only one journal publication and consequently, had very little experience writing for publication.

In spite of my frustration and disappointment in finding a commercial publisher, I was not yet ready to abandon my book project. My unrelenting desire and determination to become a published book author, led me to consider a different approach; perhaps a professional association would be a more appropriate avenue of publication. I wrote to three different associations of occupational therapy and asked if they might be interested in publishing my manuscript. This time, I sent only a query letter, introducing the subject and purpose of my book. Of the three associations I approached, one responded positively; the AOTA expressed an interest in my manuscript and requested that I forward a copy for review purposes. Following the assessment of my manuscript by two therapists, with expertise in the area of prosthetic training, the AOTA accepted to publish my manual and in February of 1980, we signed a publisher-author agreement.

Certain parts of the manuscript needed to be rewritten before the final manuscript was ready for publication. In revising the manual, I took into consideration the comments and recommendations provided not only by the two reviewers from the AOTA, but also by the 20 therapists who had originally evaluated the manual when it was part of my thesis. In addition, certain information had to be up-dated because much time had passed since the original writing; there were now new and relevant works which needed to be cited. As a result, it took another few months until the final manuscript was submitted for publication.

The AOTA made it possible for me to share my ideas and knowledge with the occupational therapists for whom my book was written. Together, we worked toward achieving the goal of publication and of contributing to the body of knowledge of our profession.

APPROACHING A PUBLISHER

In writing my first book, I experienced the joys and tribulations of book publication, and learned from my accomplishments and mistakes. Since that time, I have written several journal publications, all of which contributed to the growth and development of my writing skills. As a result, writing for publication has become a challenging, satisfying and worthwhile experience for me; I have been able to narrow the gap between my potential and my achievement as a health professional writer. Finding a publisher for my second book was much easier than the first, basically because of three important factors: (a) I chose a subject which would appeal to a profitably sized market of readers, (b) I had established my writing credibility as an author, and (c) I had a clear and organized plan for finding a publisher.

If you have an idea and material for writing a book, the following step-by-step guidelines are aimed at helping you find an appropriate publisher for your work. When approaching a publisher with an unsolicited manuscript, it is suggested that you follow four basic steps:

1. Prepare the manuscript's specifications.
2. Draw up a list of appropriate publishers to approach.
3. Select and approach one publisher.
4. Submit the manuscript's specifications to an interested publisher.

Step 1: Prepare the Manuscript's Specifications

Before approaching any publisher, it is advisable that you first prepare the manuscript's specifications, which is essentially a detailed and organized plan of your proposed book. The purpose of this document is two-fold. Firstly, it serves to develop the idea of your book; by planning the manuscript's content and format, you will begin to develop and expand upon your idea. Secondly, the manuscript's specifications provide the publisher with the initial information required to determine the publishable nature of your proposed book, as well as the estimate cost and time required to publish it.

In order that your manuscript's specifications meet both these objectives, it is suggested that you include text and format information; a table of contents; a narrative description of the chapters and professional biographical information (see Table XI).

TABLE XI
BOOK MANUSCRIPT SPECIFICATIONS

Text and Format Information
  name(s) of author(s)
  title of book
  present stage of the manuscript
  purpose and scope of the book
  primary and secondary reading audience
  technical information
  unique features of the book
  competing publications
Table of Contents
Narrative Description of the Chapters
Professional Biographical Information

Text and Format Information

In describing the text and format of your manuscript, you will need to provide the following information:

Name(s) of Author(s): Identify each of the authors by giving in full, their name; academic qualifications; official position and present affiliation; mailing address and telephone number.

Title of Book: Give the full title of the proposed book.

Present Stage of the Manuscript: Identify which of the following three stages best characterizes your manuscript:

1. Idea: You have an idea for a book, but have not yet begun writing any of the chapters.
2. Incomplete manuscript: You have written one or more chapters, but have not yet a complete manuscript.
3. Complete manuscript: You have written all the chapters of your manuscript and it is ready to be submitted for publication.

If your manuscript is in either of the first two stages of development, it is important that you indicate approximately when the manuscript will be completed.

Purpose and Scope of the Book: Provide a brief but clear description of the subject and purpose of your book. Indicate how specific or how general is the scope of the book. Explain from where the book originates; is it based on a master's thesis, doctoral dissertation, journal publication or clinical experience?

Primary and Secondary Reading Audience: Identify the reading audience to whom the book is directed. Who is the primary and the secondary reading audience? Is the book designed for a professional, student, patient or general public audience of readers? To whom will your book appeal, and if possible, explain how?

Technical Information: Give the approximate number of typewritten (double-spaced) pages, as well as the number of tables, photographs, line drawings or graphs. Specify how the manuscript will be submitted (e.g., typewritten form, on a floppy disk or on a tape).

Unique Features of the Book: Explain how your manuscript differs from any competing publications in the field. What features or particular details make it unique? Explain why these features are unique and important.

Competing Publications: Identify two or three publications in the field which would possibly compete with your work. In presenting each of these publications, be sure to include the full name of the author or editor; the year of the publication; the full title of the book; the city and name of the publisher and the price of the book.

Table of Contents

Even if your manuscript is only in the idea stage of development, it is recommended that you present to the publisher a complete table of contents. It should include not only the chapter titles and the second-place headings, but also the preliminary (e.g., foreword, preface) and end titles (e.g., references, appendix).

Narrative Description of the Chapters

To supplement the information provided in the table of contents, it is suggested that you include a narrative description of the chapters. Compose a text which explains the purpose of each chapter as well as the topics covered. Explain how the information will be presented. Will you use primarily written text or will the material be highly illustrated?

Professional Biographical Information

For each of the authors of the proposed book, it is important to present a professional biography; in addition to the information on your book, the publisher needs to know your professional experience, activities and expertise. This biographical information will serve to signify your professional competencies and your writing credibility.

The type of information which would interest the publisher includes the following:

1. Present place of employment and position.
2. Former places of employment and positions.
3. Conference presentations.
4. Research projects and grants.
5. Unpublished manuscripts.
6. Publications (e.g., books, journal articles, master's thesis or doctoral dissertation, published proceedings).

Regardless of which style or format you use to present this professional biography, be sure that the information is complete, well-organized and accurate.

Step 2: Draw Up a List of Appropriate Publishers to Approach

To determine which publishers would be most appropriate for you to approach, three important factors need to be considered: (a) the type of publisher, (b) the publisher's area of specialization, and (c) the publisher's reputation. You need first to decide which of the four types of publishers, described earlier in this chapter, will best meet your publication needs and objectives. Evaluate the advantages and disadvantages of each of these publishing options and select the one which is best for you.

It is also important to consider the subject of your manuscript in relation to the publisher's area of specialization. For example, if your topic is medical, it is advisable that you select those publishers who specialize in medical texts. On the other hand, if the focus of your manuscript is more of a professional nature, then you should consider publishers with a health publications program. Since it is necessary that the scope and purpose of your manuscript be sufficiently distinct from any other of the publisher's works, it is not recommended that you approach a publisher who has already published a book which would compete with yours.

The company's reputation is the third relevant factor to consider. You will want to select a publisher whom you regard as being reputable. For this purpose, you might want to examine some of the publishers' books and judge for yourself, the quality of these publications, in terms of their editing, design, and printing. Many publishers have available a catalog listing their publication titles and/or a brochure describing their advertising procedures; by reading through these materials, you should be able to formulate your own opinion regarding the publisher's reputation.

Taking into consideration these factors, draw up a list of potential publishers to approach.

Step 3: Select and Approach One Publisher

From your list of possible publishers, select the one you feel would best meet your publishing needs and objectives. Send a typewritten query letter, introducing your proposed book; give the full title of the manuscript and briefly describe the subject being addressed, the purpose of the proposed book, and the targeted reading audience.

The aim of this query letter is to know if the publisher you have selected, would be interested in publishing your manuscript. As Abrams (1987) notes, most publishers prefer to receive a query letter or short proposal rather than a complete manuscript. It is suggested that you write to a single publisher at a time, rather than approach several publishers at the same time. Of course, if the publisher takes too much time to decide whether or not they would be interested in your manuscript, then it might be advisable to go ahead and approach another one, rather than lose several months waiting for the first to reply.

Do not expect that the first publisher you write to will respond positively. Although it is more likely that you will receive a good many rejection letters, you only need one letter of acceptance for your book to be on its way toward publication.

Step 4: Submit the Manuscript's Specifications
to an Interested Publisher

A publisher who has responded favorably to your query letter, will request that you submit the manuscript's specifications (or in some cases, the complete manuscript) for review purposes. Therefore, it is not until you have found a publisher who is interested in your manuscript, that you need to send a detailed plan of your proposed book.

The specifications of your manuscript can be provided either by completing a specific publication data questionnaire provided by the publisher, or by preparing your own document. Regardless of the form used for your book proposal, the information to be presented will basically be that which was described earlier.

After having reviewed your manuscript's specifications, the publisher will most likely provide you with one of three types of response. Either they will agree to publish your proposed manuscript once it is completed, or they will reject it and explain why. Among the common reasons for rejection, Abrams (1987) includes the following: the subject is not worthy of book-length examination; there is no market for the subject; the book competes with a similar publication; or the book would be too expensive to publish. The third type of answer is one which is undecided; the publisher will ask to review one or more sample chapters of your manuscript, before deciding whether or not to publish your work.

Your next course of action will depend upon which of the three responses you have received. If the publisher accepts to publish your work, a publisher-author agreement will be signed, and you can begin or finish writing your manuscript. If your book proposal is rejected, you can either present the same manuscript specifications to another publisher; modify your proposal and approach another publisher; or completely abandon your book project. And lastly, if you are asked to submit one or more chapters for review, it is recommended that you do so in order that you obtain a more definite answer concerning the publishable nature of your manuscript.

PUBLISHER–AUTHOR AGREEMENT

Once you have found a publisher who has accepted to publish your book-length manuscript, you will probably be asked to sign a document titled, "publisher-author agreement." This written publishing agreement is a binding contract between you, the author, and the publisher. It serves to set forth the terms and conditions of the agreement, with regards to both parties' legal and ethical rights, responsibilities and promises. It is a necessary part of the publication process because as an author, you must know what your publisher expects of you, and what you can expect of your publisher. By clearly understanding your roles and expectations, both parties are less likely to be frustrated or disappointed.

There are various types of book-publishing contracts, however most publishers use a standard publishing agreement. Before signing this contract, it is strongly recommended that you study the entire document, reading it line by line, until you clearly understand the proposed stipulations and agreements. If you are uncertain of the meaning of certain terms, or the implications of any of the conditions, it is suggested that either you seek explanation from your publisher, or that you confer with a legal consultant (e.g., lawyer). It is your responsibility as an author, to obtain the answers to any questions you might have regarding the content of this agreement; do not hesitate to ask questions.

Although all the terms and conditions of the publisher-author agreement are important for you to consider, the following three items warrant your close attention:

1. The amount of time you have to submit the completed manuscript: Will you be able to meet this deadline?
2. The maximum number of months the publisher has to publish your book, once the submitted manuscript has been accepted: Do you consider this to be a reasonable timeframe?
3. The royalty percentage the publisher agrees to pay you: Is this percentage based on the total number of book copies sold, regardless whether or not the publisher's production costs are recovered?

QUESTIONS? ANSWERS

Question

I submitted my book-length manuscript to a publisher for review purposes. The publisher informed me that my manuscript was not suitable for publication. I am worried that since the publisher has a copy of my work, he might go ahead and publish part or all of it, without my permission. Do I have any copyright protection for my unpublished manuscript?

Answer

Yes. You are protected by federal statute against unauthorized use of your unpublished manuscript. Under the Copyright Act of 1976, which went into effect in 1978, "an original work of authorship" has copyright protection from the moment the work is in a fixed form. You own the copyright of your unpublished manuscript and all due exclusive rights, until you formally transfer copyright.

Question

Is it necessary to register my unpublished manuscript since it is automatically copyrighted from the moment it is in a fixed form? How do I proceed to have my work registered?

Answer

Although you need not register your work in order to secure copyright protection, the Copyright Office recommends that you do so, mainly for legal reasons. If your work is infringed upon, registration establishes a public record of your copyright. Also, before you can take any legal action, your work must be registered with the Copyright Office.

To register a work, simply fill out the application form provided by the Copyright Office, include a $10 fee and one copy of the work, if it is unpublished (two if published). Send this to the Register of Copyrights, Library of Congress, Washington, D.C. 20559. For information on Canadian copyright, write to Copyright and Industrial Design Branch, Place du Portage, 50 Victoria Street, Hull, Quebec, K1A 0C9.

Question

If I succeed in writing a book, and getting it published, what financial return can I expect?

Answer

Publishing a book is a very competitive and speculative venture. Although it is very difficult, if not impossible, to accurately predict how well a book will sell, several closely related factors influence the financial gain you might receive. Among them are the type of book you wrote, the number of copies sold, and the royalty percentage agreed upon. Most commercial book publishers usually agree to pay the author 10% to 15% on the retail price of each book sold. While subsidy publishers offer a higher royalty percentage (usually 40%), they require that the author pay a publishing fee; whether or not the author regains the subsidy fee, depends upon the number of book copies that are sold. Perhaps the wisest advice that can be offered on this subject is, be realistic in your expectations.

REFERENCES AND SUGGESTED READINGS

References

Abrams, D. (1987, June). Inner workings of book publishers. *Writer's Digest*, pp. 22–27.

Weiss, R. (1976). *A manual for the congenital below-elbow child amputee.* Unpublished master's thesis, Boston University, Boston.

Weiss-Lambrou, R. (1981). *A manual for the congenital unilateral below-elbow child amputee.* Rockville, MD: American Occupational Therapy Association.

Suggested Readings

Balkin, R. (1985). *How to understand & negotiate a book contract or magazine agreement.* Cincinnati, OH: Writer's Digest Books.

Bell, H. (1985). *How to get your book published: An insider's guide.* Cincinnati, OH: Writer's Digest Books.

Cool, L. C. (1987). *How to write irresistible query letters.* Cincinnati, OH: Writer's Digest Books.

Larsen, M. (1985). *How to write a book proposal.* Cincinnati, OH: Writer's Digest Books.

Patton, W. L. (1980). *An author's guide to the copyright law.* Lexington, MA: Lexington Books.

Polking, K. (1987). *A beginner's guide to getting published.* Cincinnati, OH: Writer's Digest Books.

Ross, T., & Ross, M. (1985). *The complete guide to self-publishing.* Cincinnati, OH: Writer's Digest Books.

Steich, T. J. (1982). What the copyright laws mean to the writer. *American Journal of Occupational Therapy, 36,* 604–606.

Chapter V

FROM START TO FINISH

There must be a beginning of any great matter, but the continuing unto the end until it be thoroughly finished yields the true glory.
Sir Francis Drake

The task of writing for publication is not easy, especially for the novice health professional writer. It requires good writing skills as well as such attitudinal competencies as motivation, perseverance and self-discipline. The health professional who aspires to become a published author can acquire these qualifications and learn to write successfully for publication. Many health professionals however, do not become published authors because they have difficulty beginning and/or completing their manuscript. This is understandable because it is just as difficult to start as it is to finish writing.

For the purpose of learning to write successfully for publication, this chapter provides suggestions on how to start and finish writing a manuscript. It also presents ten basic steps to writing for publication and summarily explains how the typewritten manuscript is transmuted into the printed page.

SUGGESTIONS FOR GETTING STARTED

To help you get started on the road to publication, the following three suggestions are offered: select a realistic writing project; apply the fundamentals of writing for publication; and begin with the "write" attitude.

Select a Realistic Writing Project

In writing for publication, it is of critical importance that you choose a realistic writing project; you need to select the type of manuscript which you will be able to write best. So many novice writers are overwhelmed by the size of their project that they have much difficulty beginning to write. Also, once they do begin to write, they tend to focus on the quantity of work to be done rather than on the quality of their writing.

In order to determine which type of manuscript would be the most appropriate and perhaps the easiest to write as your first publication, it is suggested that you consider the pyramid of writing for publication, presented in Figure 2.

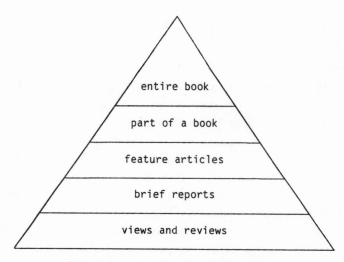

Figure 2. Pyramid of writing for publication.

According to this pyramid, there are five levels of publication for the health professional writer. Views and reviews are at the bottom of the pyramid because the format of this type of paper is relatively simple. Also, the length of the manuscript is very short and as such, generally requires a small amount of time to complete. Writing a letter to the editor or a book review will provide you with some writing experience and help you acquire confidence in your ability to put words on paper.

The second level of publication is comprised of brief reports. Manuscripts of this kind are a good training ground for later writing a feature article or book. Because this manuscript is short, you can write it in a relatively small amount of time. This is not to say that writing a brief report is easy. All good writing is demanding, particularly the brief report, because its distinct length demands that you be as succinct and as clear as possible; there is no room for verbose text or lengthy descriptions. Just like a short story, a brief report must be of excellent quality if it is to succeed in this form.

Feature articles constitute the third level of writing for publication. Because of the nature and style of this type of manuscript, writing a good feature article requires that you be able to analyze, organize and synthesize a large number of works; to report published information clearly and accurately; and to discuss issues in an objective, but yet critical, perspective. This type of publication is an excellent experience for later writing a book; the content of one or more feature articles can serve as a foundation for a future book publication.

The fourth level of the pyramid involves writing part of a book. If you aspire to become a book author, but do not feel that you could cope with the size of such a writing project, you might consider writing a book with one or two other persons, or contributing to a book publication by writing a chapter. Although this type of writing project is exacting in terms of time and effort, it is advantageous as you are not alone in your writing. The other authors or the book editor can support and encourage you; share with you their ideas, knowledge and experiences; and provide you with constructive criticism.

Writing an entire book by yourself, is the fifth and highest level of writing for publication. To successfully become a book author, you must have the utmost qualifications; you must excel not only in your knowledge on the subject, but also in your writing skills and in your attitudinal competencies. Because you are the sole author, a publication of this kind is very demanding in terms of the effort and time you must expend in writing the book and in finding a publisher. The satisfaction and pleasure gained however, from having a book published, makes this type of writing project perhaps the most challenging and worthwhile accomplishment as a health professional author.

Although the pyramid ranks the types of manuscripts according to degree of difficulty, it is meant to be viewed only as a guideline for helping you to begin writing for publication; it is not intended to propose that one level is an absolute pre-requisite for the next. If you want to become a published author, begin by selecting a realistic writing project; begin at the bottom of the pyramid, not at the top. In this way, you will develop your writing skills, acquire valuable writing experience, and succeed in writing for publication.

Apply the Fundamentals of Writing for Publication

Many novice health professional writers either do not know the fundamentals of writing for publication or do not know how to apply them when writing. As a result, they have much difficulty beginning their manuscript. Writing for publication is something that can be learned, acquired, and mastered. You should not begin to write unless you understand the basic principles and are determined to apply them in your writing. For example, many novice health professional writers fail to recognize that not all manuscripts are written the same way. As explained in Chapter III, each type of manuscript has its own writing style and component parts; a mixture of styles is extremely undesirable. By reading, understanding and applying the fundamentals of writing for publication, as presented in this book, you will be able to embark on an auspicious journey to publication.

Begin with the "Write" Attitude

Your attitude both as a health professional and as a writer are critical to successfully writing for publication. It is strongly recommended that you begin with the "write" attitude.

Be confident in your ability to write. Be motivated and stay motivated to achieve your goal. Be goal-oriented. Be determined to do the best you can. Be resourceful in your finding and setting aside time to write. Be creative in your thoughts and ideas. Be objective and professional in your writing. Be open and receptive to criticism. By beginning with the "write" attitude, you will develop your aptitude as a writer and your potential as a published author.

SUGGESTIONS FOR GETTING FINISHED

"When will you finish writing?" This was the question I was most frequently asked during the time I wrote this book. It seems that people were generally more interested in when the manuscript would be completed than when it was started, or even, why I was writing a book. Although this question sometimes made me anxious, especially if it was asked more than one time in a week, it nonetheless led me to include in this section, two important guidelines to getting finished: know when to stop writing and how to add the finishing touches to your manuscript.

When to Stop Writing

It is not easy to know when a manuscript is finished and ready to be submitted for review. The novice writer often has difficulty determining the final version of the manuscript. How much rewriting is necessary before the manuscript should be submitted? How much rewriting is necessary for the manuscript to meet the criteria for publication?

In the writer's desire to finish the manuscript, one of two problems often occurs. First, the manuscript is submitted for review but does not meet the criteria for publication; it is judged as requiring further rewriting and consequently, is not accepted as submitted. Second, in an attempt to write the "perfect" paper, the writer is unable to complete the manuscript and as a result, never submits it for review.

To overcome both of these problems, it is suggested that you critically evaluate your manuscript. If you feel that it has potential for being published, even though it may not be "perfect," submit it for review. Do not write on endlessly; abandon your search for perfection or else you will never finish. Do not be a writer of unpublished manuscripts; finish what you started and do not fear criticism. The outcome of the review process will determine the publishable nature of your manuscript. Knowing when and being able to stop writing is an important part of bringing your manuscript to completion.

How to Add the Finishing Touches

Once you have finished writing your manuscript, you need to add some final touches, before submitting it for review. This involves following the journal's guidelines to presenting and submitting your manuscript; preparing the title page of your manuscript; writing a covering letter; and obtaining any required letters of permission and consent.

Before submitting your work for review, you need to be certain that you have followed the journal's instructions for presenting and submitting your manuscript. Most journals require that the work be typed, double-spaced (including references, legends and footnotes), on standard (8½″ × 11″) white bond paper, with one inch margins on all four sides. The entire manuscript should be numbered consecutively, beginning with the title page. You need to submit the original, plus the required number of photocopies (usually three or four). For the purpose of a blind review, the manuscript copies should not include any identification of the author(s).

If you have not done so as yet, prepare the title page of your manuscript. The information to be included on this page is as follows: the title of the manuscript; the full name of the author(s); a footnote of biographical data for each author (i.e., academic qualifications, official position and present affiliation); and a footnote if the work was supported by a grant or originates from a master's thesis, doctoral dissertation or conference presentation. In addition, many health professional journals request that a certain number of key words (usually two or three) be identified on the title page; these key words should reflect the subject being addressed and will be used for indexing purposes.

A covering or transmittal letter, addressed to the editor, must accompany your manuscript. The purpose of this letter is to request review and possible publication of your manuscript. It should be well-written, neatly typed and signed by all authors. Although the information that must be contained in the covering letter will vary, depending upon each journal's specifications, it generally includes the following:

1. The title of the manuscript.
2. The name(s) of the author(s).
3. The name, address and telephone number of the author to whom all correspondence should be sent.
4. A statement attesting that the work is original and has not been previously published elsewhere.
5. A statement attesting that the undersigned author or authors are the sole owners of the submitted work.
6. A statement attesting that the submitted manuscript is not under concurrent consideration for publication elsewhere.
7. A statement assigning all copyright ownership to the publisher.

With reference to this last point, it is to be understood that if the manuscript is accepted for publication, the authors agree to assign their literary rights to the publisher, via a copyright release form. Some journals request that the authors sign this form when submitting their manuscript for review, while others ask that it be signed only if and when the manuscript has been accepted for publication.

If you have included any copyrighted material in your manuscript, you need to provide for the editor, evidence that permission to reprint was granted from the copyright owner. In other words, written permission from the copyright source must be obtained to quote at length textual matter and to reproduce or adapt, all or part of a table or a figure, taken from a previously published work. Also, if your manuscript includes photographs of any identifiable persons, you need to obtain (from the subject, parent, or guardian) written consent to use the photographs in your publication.

In summary, when submitting your manuscript for review, you need to include the original copy of your manuscript, plus the required number of photocopies; a covering letter; and any required letters of permission or consent. This entire manuscript packet should be properly parceled, so that it be protected from any possible damage during mailing. Because the journal is not responsible for the loss of any manuscripts, it is strongly recommended that you keep at least one copy of all materials you have submitted.

TEN BASIC STEPS TO WRITING FOR PUBLICATION

To help the health professional writer achieve the goal of publication, this section describes ten basic steps (see Table XII) in writing a journal or book-length manuscript; this step-by-step approach is a synthesis of the writing principles explained in this book. If followed closely and correctly, this "write" approach will simplify the writing process and maximize the manuscript's publishing potential.

TABLE XII
TEN BASIC STEPS TO WRITING FOR PUBLICATION

From start	1. Select a realistic writing project
	2. Identify the topic
	3. Determine the purpose of the manuscript
	4. Choose the most appropriate publisher
	5. Plan your work
	6. Read and write
	7. Reread and rewrite
	8. Conform to the publisher's guidelines
	9. Submit the manuscript for review
to finish	10. Revise the manuscript

Step 1: Select a Realistic Writing Project

The first and perhaps the most important step of writing for publication is selecting a realistic writing project. As explained earlier in this chapter, the pyramid of writing for publication can be used as a guideline to helping you determine which type of manuscript to write. Exercise discrimination and select the writing project, you will be able to write best.

In order to make the right choice, you must of course know your abilities and your limitations. Are you able to write independently or do you need support and guidance from co-authors? Do you have the self-discipline, motivation and perseverance needed for this type of writing project? Are your writing goals realistic? If necessary, are you willing to use your personal time for writing some or all of the manuscript?

Step 2: Identify the Topic

The topic you select must be one for which you are qualified to write. It should also be a timely topic and one that contributes to the knowledge and practice of the targeted reading audience. Do you have the knowledge, clinical experience and expertise on the subject? Is the type of manuscript you have selected the most appropriate for writing on this topic? What is the nature and scope of the topic? Is the subject too broad or too narrow? How will your manuscript differ from other publications that have addressed the same or similar topic?

For the health professional writer, there are so many topics to choose from, but yet so little time to write. Because your time is so valuable, be sure to choose a topic that is worth writing, publishing, and reading.

Step 3: Determine the Purpose of the Manuscript

To determine the purpose of your manuscript, you need to identify the reading audience for whom the manuscript is intended and the reason(s) for writing the manuscript. Who is the targeted primary and secondary reading audience? Are you addressing a professional, student, or general public audience of readers? What is your purpose for writing? How will the publication be of value and of interest to the readers?

It is important to remember that the clearer the work's purpose is for you, the clearer it will be for the reviewers assessing your manuscript and for the readers reading your publication.

Step 4: Choose the Most Appropriate Publisher

Bearing in mind the type of manuscript you have selected, the topic you are addressing, and the purpose for writing the manuscript, you now need to determine the journal or book publisher to whom your work will be submitted. Which publisher would best meet your publication needs and objectives? Which publisher do you think would be interested in your manuscript?

To help you make this decision, it is strongly recommended that you examine recent publications of several different publishers. If you are writing a journal manuscript, study recent issues of various journals; examine the tables of content, guidelines for authors, and the content and writing style of the publications. What types of articles are featured? Who is the primary reading audience of the journal? Is the journal peer-reviewed? Is it considered to be a prestigious journal? How frequently is the journal published? Although you may have more than one journal in mind, narrow down your choice to one; it is unethical to simultaneously submit your manuscript to more than one journal.

If you are writing a book manuscript, examine the publications of several different book publishers. What type of publisher should you select? What is the publisher's area of specialization? What types of books or subjects are featured? Who is the primary and secondary reading audience of these books? Is the publisher considered to be reputable? Select the publisher who you feel would be the most appropriate for your manuscript.

Step 5: Plan Your Work

In writing any type of manuscript for publication, it is necessary that you carefully plan your time and your writing (see "The Writing Process" in Chap. I). This involves preparing a well-drawn outline of your manuscript, gathering the information you will need for writing, and determining a realistic writing schedule.

How will the manuscript be organized? What are the component parts of the manuscript? What headings and sub-headings will be most appropriate for these parts? How much time will be required to write the manuscript? Is your time plan realistic? How do you plan on obtaining your information?

So many novice health professional writers do not realize the importance of planning their work, and as a result, submit manuscripts that are hastily and poorly, planned and written. The number of hours spent writing is not necessarily a measure of the quality of your writing, nor is it a reason for justifying that your manuscript be published. Often, too much time is spent writing because of poor planning. If you take the time to properly plan your work, not only will you save much time and effort, but more importantly, you will produce a manuscript of maximum quality and value.

Step 6: Read and Write

Reading and writing go hand in hand, and for this reason, are presented together as the next step to writing for publication. To become a published author, you must be a reader and a writer. The more you read, the better reader you will become; the more you write, the better writer you will become; the more you read and write, the greater your potential in becoming a published author.

What should you read? Read what other health professionals have written. If you are writing a clinical report, read published clinical reports, especially in recent issues of the journal to which your manuscript will be submitted. Similarly, if you are writing a research article, read published research articles. Reading recent publications that are similar to your topic or to the type of manuscript you have selected, will help you to develop and improve your writing skills; study the content, writing style, length and format of these publications. Use these works as a model for learning to write for publication.

How should you write? Apply the principles of writing for publication and write as best you can. If necessary, begin in note form. Develop your notes into sentences, then into paragraphs. Connect one paragraph to the next. Logically develop the transition from one part of the manuscript to the next. Remember that you are writing for a particular reading audience; your language level must be appropriate to this audience.

Step 7: Reread and Rewrite

Once you have written a good preliminary draft of your manuscript, reread your work to determine what needs to be rewritten. The purpose of rewriting is to improve the manuscript's quality in terms of its content and writing style (see "The Writing Process" in Chap.I). In order for your manuscript to meet the criteria for publication, you need to reread and rewrite. You should stop rewriting only when you feel that your manuscript has potential for being published and is ready to be submitted for review.

In rewriting your manuscript, be sure that your writing is concise, precise and logically organized. Verify that your information is complete, meaningful and accurate. Check for typographical, grammatical, spelling and punctuation errors. Evaluate your manuscript critically and rewrite, until it is just "write."

Step 8: Conform to the Publisher's Guidelines

Most health professional journals and book publishers provide, for prospective authors, guidelines to presenting and submitting a manuscript. A large number of manuscripts submitted for review, clearly reveal that the writer did not follow the publisher's guidelines. This is a serious, frequent and unnecessary problem. Why risk having your manuscript rejected for this reason, when the publisher specifies how it should be prepared? Just reading these instructions is not enough; you must follow them exactly. You must prepare your manuscript the publisher's way, not your way. In writing for publication, there are numerous rules which must be respected; many principles which must be applied; but one editorial style which must be adopted. It is of paramount importance that your manuscript conforms to the style adopted by the journal or book publisher to whom your work will be submitted. Close adherence to the guidelines will maximize the manuscript's publishing potential.

Step 9: Submit the Manuscript for Review

All manuscripts written for publication in a peer-reviewed journal, are submitted to the editor for review purposes. It is necessary to include the following documents: the original manuscript, plus the required number of photocopies; a covering letter requesting review and possible publication of the manuscript; and any required letters of permission or consent. When a manuscript has been received, the editor usually writes to the designated correspondent author and acknowledges receipt of the submitted manuscript. To determine its suitability for publication, the work will then be reviewed by the journal reviewers selected by the editor. The length of time required for the review process varies with each journal, however, it usually takes two to three months (American Psychological Association, 1983).

If you have written a book manuscript, it is suggested that you approach a publisher by first sending a query letter (see "Approaching a Publisher" in Chap.IV). The manuscript's specifications should be submitted for review only when a publisher has manifested an interest in your book idea. Usually, the final or complete manuscript is submitted after a publisher-author agreement has been signed.

Step 10: Revise the Manuscript

The review of any type of manuscript, generally results in one of four outcomes: (a) The manuscript is accepted as submitted; (b) the manuscript is accepted, conditional upon minor or moderate revisions; (c) the manuscript is unacceptable as submitted and requires major revisions; and (d) the manuscript is rejected. Thus, the last and final step to writing for publication will depend upon which of these four recommendations you received.

If your manuscript was accepted as submitted, you should consider yourself an exceptional writer; Day (1979) reports that only 5% of the manuscripts submitted to journals are accepted as presented. Because your manuscript does not require any revisions, you can omit this last step and proceed with processing your work for publication.

If your manuscript was accepted, conditional upon minor or moderate revisions, you must complete the tenth step; revise your manuscript in compliance with the reviewers' comments, suggestions and recommendations. Do not rewrite those parts of your manuscript that have been judged as being acceptable because you may create new problems; concentrate on making the requested changes. Resubmit the revised manuscript for review. Most journals specify the maximum amount of time (usually six months) that will be allowed for submitting the revised manuscript; failure to respect this deadline can result in the manuscript being rejected.

If your manuscript was found to be unacceptable in its present form, thereby requiring major revisions, you need to revise your manuscript accordingly. In this case, because the revisions are considered to be major, some parts or all of the manuscript will require much rewriting. Evaluate your work critically, in light of the reviewers' comments and criticisms. Do not be discouraged; persevere in improving your manuscript. Resubmit your manuscript for review and explain, in a covering letter, what revisions have been made.

If your manuscript was rejected, do not feel that you are alone; more than 50% of the manuscripts submitted to journals are rejected (Bishop, 1981; Day, 1979). What can you do when your manuscript has not been accepted for publication? Basically, you have one of three options: (a) Submit the same manuscript to another journal; (b) revise the manuscript and submit it to another journal; and (c) abandon your writing project. Because most journals usually explain why a manuscript has been rejected, it is advisable that you base your next course of action on the reason(s) given. For example, if the topic of your manuscript was found to be unsuitable for the journal's readers, then you should consider submitting the same manuscript to a more appropriate journal. On the other hand, if your manuscript was rejected because it was poorly organized and written, you need to determine whether or not you want to revise and submit it to another journal. Abandoning your writing project is not encouraged, unless you no longer have the desire or motivation to have your manuscript published. Provided that you are able to recognize where, how and why you failed in your writing, you should try again.

If you have followed these ten basic steps and your manuscript has been accepted for publication, you can now proceed with the publisher, to getting your work into print and to becoming a published author.

GETTING INTO PRINT

Getting into print refers to the publication or production processing of an accepted manuscript. There are several stages of production, each of which involve the combined efforts and expertise of many persons; to name but a few, they include the publisher, editor, associate editor, managing editor, copy editor, production manager, printer, design and art director, and of course, the author. Although the policies and procedures for processing an accepted manuscript can vary with each journal or book publisher, it is important for the health professional writer to have a basic understanding of how the typewritten manuscript is transmuted into the printed page. For this purpose, this section summarily outlines the publication process.

The accepted manuscript is first subjected to copy-editing, which involves line-by-line editing by the editor and/or copy editor. Editorial changes to the accepted manuscript largely consist of correction of spelling, punctuation, and grammar, and the improvement of consistency of style or clarity of expression.

Photocopies of the copy-edited manuscript are usually sent to the designated correspondent author for review and approval. The author is responsible for revising, condensing or correcting any material and for answering any of the copy editor's questions. The reviewed and approved copy-edited manuscript must be returned to the editorial office, within a specified period of time so as not to delay the next steps of production. The copy-edited manuscript is then sent to the printer for typesetting.

After the manuscript is set into type, the typeset proofs need to be critically read and checked for any typographical errors; this stage of the publication process is referred to as the proof stage. Usually it is the author who is responsible for the critical reading of the proofs, however, not all journals send the proofs to the author; in some cases, the journal's editorial staff assumes this responsibility. Standard proofreaders' marks are used to indicate any changes on the proofs. Only corrections of typographical errors should be made at this time; any other alterations are not desirable and the author may be charged for any such changes. This is why it is so important that the author make any necessary changes when reviewing the copy-edited manuscript, rather than when proofreading. The corrected proofs must be promptly returned to the editorial office so as to eliminate any delay in publication. These proofs are then prepared into page layouts, and the final product is the printed page.

How quickly a manuscript is transformed into print depends on various factors such as, the type of publication; the topic and the length of the manuscript; the amount of time required for editing, proofreading, design and production; the priority for publication; and the publication schedule of the publisher. According to the American Psychological Association (1983), the publication lag, or the time interval between the date an accepted journal manuscript is received in an editor's office and the date the manuscript is published, usually does not exceed 12 months.

For a manuscript to travel the long road of publication, both the author and the journal or book publisher's staff must work in close collaboration. It is only then that the goal of publication can be successfully achieved.

In closing this book, I wish to leave you with this:

As a health professional, you have a certain obligation
To disseminate new knowledge through publication.
In order to achieve this goal, it is essential
To develop your writing and publishing potential.
With the "write" approach and attitude,
Learn to maximize your writing aptitude.
Begin writing your journal or book manuscript today
And become a published author without further delay.

QUESTIONS? ANSWERS

Question

As a novice health professional writer, I am somewhat worried about the criticism I will receive from my peers; I have difficulty completing my manuscript because I fear the outcome of the peer review. Do health professionals, who have had several articles published, also fear such criticism?

Answer

For the novice health professional writer, fear of criticism from one's peers is a common emotional barrier to writing for publication. In order for you to finish writing, you must try to overcome this problem by recognizing that the peer review process is a means of helping you to improve the quality of your manuscript.

Based on my experience as a journal reviewer, I have found that although most experienced health professional writers do not fear criticism, some tend to have difficulty accepting it. That is, some (not all) health professional writers feel that because they have had several publications, their manuscript will be readily accepted as submitted; when faced with the reviewers' recommendation that their manuscript be revised, they become insulted or even resentful.

Being unable to accept criticism is perhaps just as great a barrier to getting published as is fear of criticism. Regardless of whether you are a new or an experienced writer, the "write" attitude implies that you be receptive to your peer's assessment of your manuscript and that you act upon these recommendations accordingly. Once your work is published, you must also be able to accept any criticism you might receive from the readers of your publication.

Question

I realize that it is difficult, if not impossible, for you to estimate how much time would be involved in my writing a journal manuscript, from start to finish. As a point of reference for me, how long does it take for you to write and publish a journal article?

Answer

There are many factors that influence the amount of time invested in a publication, for example, the type of manuscript, the writing experience of the writer(s), the time available for writing, and the outcome of the review process. Because of these variables, it is difficult to make a general statement as to how long it would take for any health professional, myself included, to write and publish a journal article. However, since you would like a point of reference, I will give you a concrete example.

In June 1987, I began to write a research article, in collaboration with two co-authors. The completed manuscript was submitted for review in December of that year. We were informed of the outcome of the review process in March 1988; the manuscript was accepted, conditional upon minor revisions. We revised the manuscript as requested and resubmitted it in May 1988. It was officially accepted for publication in August and was published in October 1988.

As you can see, even for a health professional with writing experience, much time is involved in the writing and publication process; it took almost one and a half years, from the time we started the manuscript to the time it was published. I consider this to be a reasonable period of time, considering the factors which influenced our writing project.

Question

With reference to the pyramid of writing for publication, you suggest that for a first publication, the novice health professional writer should begin at the bottom of the pyramid, rather than at the top. As I understand, you wrote an entire book, after having had only one journal publication. Could you please explain why you did not follow the hierarchy of the pyramid.

Answer

The pyramid of writing for publication is the outgrowth of my experience both as an author and journal reviewer. When I decided to write my first book, I did not discriminate between the different types of manuscripts. My choice was based primarily on my desire and determination to become a book author, rather than on my understanding and application of the principles of writing for publication. Although I succeeded in achieving my goal, I made several mistakes in the process, encountered many difficulties that could have been avoided, and lost much valuable time and effort. I believe that it is so much easier to write for publication, when one has some clear guidelines as to where and how to begin; this is why and how I came to conceive the pyramid of writing for publication.

REFERENCES AND SUGGESTED READINGS

References

American Psychological Association. (1983). *Publication manual of the American Psychological Association* (3rd ed.). Washington, DC: Author.

Bishop, B. (1981). Contents of a paper for presentation. *Physiotherapy Canada, 33,* 277–280.

Day, R. A. (1979). *How to write and publish a scientific paper.* Philadelphia, PA: ISI Press.

Suggested Readings

Cleather, J. (1981). Manuscript review and the editing process. *Physiotherapy Canada, 33,* 283–286.

Plotnik, A. (1982). *The elements of editing: A modern guide for editors and journalists.* New York: Macmillan.

Skillin, M. E., & Gay, R. M. (1974). *Words into type* (3rd ed.). Englewood Cliffs, NJ: Prentice-Hall.

University of Chicago Press. (1982). *The Chicago manual of style* (13th ed., rev.). Chicago: Author.

Wall, J. (1974). Getting into print in P & G: How it's done. *Personnel and Guidance Journal, 52,* 594–602.

LIST OF JOURNALS IN THE HEALTH FIELD

NURSING

American Journal of Nursing
Canadian Nurse
Dimensions of Critical Care Nursing
Journal of Gerontological Nursing
Journal of Nursing Administration
Nurse Educator
Nursing
Nursing Management
Nursing Outlook
Nursing Research
Rehabilitation Nursing

OCCUPATIONAL THERAPY

American Journal of Occupational Therapy
Australian Occupational Therapy Journal
British Journal of Occupational Therapy
Canadian Journal of Occupational Therapy
Occupational Therapy in Health Care
Occupational Therapy in Mental Health
Occupational Therapy Journal of Research
Physical & Occupational Therapy in Geriatrics
Physical & Occupational Therapy in Pediatrics

PHYSICAL MEDICINE AND REHABILITATION

American Archives of Rehabilitation Therapy
American Journal of Physical Medicine
American Rehabilitation

Archives of Physical Medicine and Rehabilitation
British Journal of Rheumatology
British Journal of Sports Medicine
Canadian Journal of Rehabilitation
Cognitive Rehabilitation
International Journal of Rehabilitation Research
International Rehabilitation Medicine
Journal of Applied Rehabilitation Counseling
Journal of Rehabilitation
Journal of Rehabilitation Research and Development
Rehabilitation Digest
Rehabilitation Gazette
Rehabilitation Literature
Rehabilitation World
Rheumatology and Rehabilitation
Scandinavian Journal of Rehabilitation Medicine

PHYSICAL THERAPY

Australian Journal of Physiotherapy
Clinical Management in Physical Therapy
Journal of Orthopaedic and Sports Physical Therapy
Physical & Occupational Therapy in Geriatrics
Physical & Occupational Therapy in Pediatrics
Physical Therapy
Physical Therapy in Health Care
Physiotherapy
Physiotherapy Canada

PSYCHOLOGY

American Psychologist
Contemporary Psychology
Developmental Psychology
Journal of Abnormal Psychology
Journal of Applied Psychology
Journal of Comparative Psychology
Journal of Consulting and Clinical Psychology
Journal of Counseling Psychology

Journal of Educational Psychology
Journal of Experimental Psychology: General
Journal of Experimental Psychology: Learning, Memory and Cognition
Journal of Experimental Psychology: Human Perception and Performance
Journal of Personality and Social Psychology
Professional Psychology: Research and Practice
Psychological Bulletin
Psychological Review

SOCIAL WORK

Administration in Social Work
Journal of Gerontological Social Work
Health and Social Work
Social Work in Health Care
Social Work with Groups

SPEECH AND AUDIOLOGY

ASHA: Journal of the American Speech and Hearing Association
Journal of Speech and Hearing Disorders
Journal of Speech and Hearing Research
Hearing Journal
Hearing Research
Speech Technology

JOURNALS OF RELATED INTEREST

Activities, Adaptation & Aging
Biofeedback and Self-Regulation
Brain
Brain and Cognition
Brain and Language
Canadian Journal of Community Mental Health
Clinical Gerontologist
Clinical Prosthetics and Orthotics
Dimensions in Health Service
Ergonomics
Geriatrics

Health Care in Canada
Health Care Management Review
Home Health Care Services Quarterly
Journal of Allied Health
Journal of Biomechanics
Journal of Gerontology
Journal of Psychosocial Oncology
Journal of Women & Aging
New England Journal of Medicine
Orthotics and Prosthetics
Prosthetics and Orthotics International
Research on Aging
Sexuality and Disability
The Hospice Journal
Women & Health

Appendix B

MANUSCRIPT REVIEW FORMS

Appendix B.1

AMERICAN JOURNAL OF OCCUPATIONAL THERAPY*

Date:

Manuscript:

Please review and discuss the enclosed manuscript in terms of:

- the appropriateness and timeliness of the subject matter for the AJOT audience (new approach, development of theory)
- the soundness of the approach (of the program or of the research design)
- are implications for occupational therapy clearly stated?
- the quality of the text in terms of clarity, logical development, conciseness, and readability
- the quality of the data presentation (charts, graphs, tables)

Return your comments within two weeks from the above date. If the manuscript requires revision, please be specific in your recommendations. Your assistance is quite helpful to the author and the editor. Sincere thanks for your reviews.

The following checklist is provided for summarizing your reactions:

Value of topic for readers

_____ Excellent _____ Very Good _____ Good _____ Fair _____ Poor

A. Accept as is   _____

B. Revision required   _____

   Condense   _____

   Rewrite   _____

   Add data   _____

   Reorganize   _____

---

*Reprinted with permission from the American Occupational Therapy Association, Inc.

Re-do charts/tables   ————————
C. Reject   ————————
    Unoriginal   ————————
    Poorly written   ————————
    Unwarranted conclusions   ————————
    Insufficient importance   ————————
    Other   ————————
D. Comments

ARCHIVES OF PHYSICAL MEDICINE AND REHABILITATION*

Manuscript Review

Manuscript Title: _____

_____

Author(s): _____

Primary Reviewer: _____

Telephone Number: _____(_____)_____

INSTRUCTIONS

As you review this manuscript, please concern yourself primarily with its content and not its style (i.e., do not be concerned with correct reference form, etc.). You may write comments and observations on this copy of the manuscript, if it will help you in making a judgement about the paper. Please remember that the section editor is relying upon your *critical* evaluation, so be as thorough as possible when you complete the attached comment sheet. When you have finished your review, mail all materials to the section editor in the enclosed envelope. We appreciate your *prompt* review of this manuscript and your cooperation in agreeing to review it. Please do not sign your REVIEWER COMMENT sheet. Sign only this sheet and return it *with* the comment sheet.

RECOMMENDATION

This article should be: _____ Accepted as submitted
                        _____ Rejected

_____ Accepted subject to revisions
specified.

NAME (typed or printed)	DATE

SIGNATURE

Primary Reviewer Comment Sheet
for
The Archives of Physical Medicine and Rehabilitation

Manuscript Title: _____

_____

Author(s): _____

(Please type or print your comments.)

INTRODUCTION: (Does it adequately state the purpose and rationale
for the study as well as the methodology?)

EXPERIMENTAL DESIGN OF THE STUDY: (Is it adequate?)

METHODS: (Please comment here, if appropriate, on the statistical
method)

RESULTS: (Are results derived from the experimental design and the
statistics?)

DISCUSSION:

SUMMARY:

ABSTRACT:

FIGURES:

REFERENCES: (If you are acquainted with relevant literature not cited in this manuscript, please cite it here.)

(NOTE: PLEASE USE ADDITIONAL SHEETS, WHERE NECESSARY, TO COMPLETE YOUR REVIEW.)

Appendix B.3

CANADIAN JOURNAL OF
OCCUPATIONAL THERAPY*

Manuscript—General Checklist

REVIEWER _____ MANUSCRIPT # _____

_____

_____

	Yes	No
Logical flow of ideas	_____	_____
Clear and precise language	_____	_____
Key terms defined	_____	_____
Non-sexist language	_____	_____
Accurate referencing A.P.A. style	_____	_____
All references present in reference list	_____	_____
Clearly stated assumptions, rationale	_____	_____
Tables & figures complement, not duplicate text	_____	_____
Conclusions and implications clear	_____	_____
Well-organised and well-written	_____	_____
Appropriate length	_____	_____

RECOMMENDATIONS

1. Accept as is _____ Yes / *No*

2/3 Revisions required: Major   Minor   Optional   4. Reject _____

	Major	Minor	Optional	
Condense	_____	_____	_____	Unoriginal ____
Add	_____	_____	_____	Poorly written
Reorganise				
Re-do figs/tables	_____	_____	_____	_____
_____	_____	_____	_____	
_____	_____	_____	_____	
_____	_____	_____	_____	

Canadian Journal of Occupational Therapy
Manuscript Evaluation Form

RESEARCH ARTICLES

REVIEWER _____ MANUSCRIPT # _____

_____

_____

Abstract

Title

Introduction

Literature Review

Methodology

Results

Discussion

Conclusion

Figures & Tables

References

JOURNAL OF ALLIED HEALTH*

Number _____

Title _____

Reviewer _____ Date Sent _____ Date Back _____

Content appropriate to Journal _____ no _____ yes

Recommendation

Accept (no revisions) _____ Accept (minor revisions) _____

Provisionally accept pending major revisions, return for second review

_____

Reject _____ Reviewers Signature _____

Title of Article: _____ Acceptable as is
                         _____ Inappropriate, should read: _____
                         _____

Abstract: _____ Acceptable as is _____ Too long
                         _____ Does not accurately reflect the text

Subheadings: _____ Appropriate
                         _____ Inappropriate to section content,
                                       should read: _____
                         _____

Methodology: _____ Appropriate for this type of study
                         _____ Inappropriate for this type of study,
                                       should have applied the following: __
                         _____

Tables and Figures: _____ All acceptable
                         _____ The following should be deleted or
                                       revised:_____
                         _____

---

*Developed by the editorial office of the Journal of Allied Health and reprinted with permission from the Journal of Allied Health.

References:

_____	Acceptable as is	_____	Current
_____	In AMA Style	_____	Not current
_____	Not in AMA style,	_____	Too many
	need to be revised	_____	Too few
			(literature search inadequate)

In comparison with other articles of similar content, scope, and approach, this manuscript is:

_____ Superior   _____ Below Average

_____ Above Average   _____ Poor

_____ Average

USE OPPOSITE SIDE TO MAKE COMMENTS TO AUTHORS REGARDING CONTENT AND STYLE

Appendix B.5

JOURNAL OF NURSING ADMINISTRATION AND NURSE EDUCATOR*

Suzanne Smith Blancett, RN, EdD
   Editor-in-Chief
210 Daniel Webster Highway South
Suite #4
Nashua, NH 03060
   [603] 888-2530

( ) THE JOURNAL OF NURSING
   ADMINISTRATION
( ) NURSE EDUCATOR
MANUSCRIPT REVIEW FORM

REVIEWER _____ DATE _____

MS. TITLE _____

It's most helpful to me, and the authors, if, as you read, you write your spontaneous positive, negative, and developmental comments right on the manuscript pages. Return only the marked pages along with this form.

	YES	NO	COMMENT
Does the paper present new findings or ideas?			
If no, does it present old material better?			
Is the content clearly presented, without jargon?			
Is the content sophisticated enough for our readers?			
Is the content timely/relevant?			
Will the paper be outdated/unimportant if published in 8–12 months?			
Introduction—Is the purpose of the paper clear?			
Methods			
• Is the sample and sampling method adequate?			
• Are data collection instruments reliable and valid?			
• Are statistical tests appropriate?			
Are references recent and relevant?			
Does the author draw conclusions/generalizations beyond what findings/data/arguments support?			
Is the application or usefulness of the content made explicit to the reader's practice setting?			

*Reprinted with permission from the Journal of Nursing Administration & Nurse Educator, 1988, J. B. Lippincott Company, Philadelphia, Pennsylvania.

138

Is the content logically and clearly developed? _____ _____
Was the paper interesting to read? _____ _____

RECOMMENDATION:
( ) PUBLISH   ( ) PUBLISH AFTER REVISION   ( ) REJECT
GENERAL COMMENTS/SUGGESTIONS: (Please print or type. Use reverse side
                                                        if necessary.)

Appendix B.6

REHABILITATION NURSING*

Manuscript Review Form

Manuscript number: _____

Please review this manuscript with respect to its suitability for publication in *Rehabilitation Nursing*. Return this form within three (3) weeks, but no later than _____. Do *not* return the manuscript; it should be destroyed. REMEMBER: An unpublished manuscript is the sole property of the author(s) and should be treated as such. If you are unable to meet the deadline for return of your review, please notify me immediately!

1. My recommendation is:
   _____ Accept for publication
   _____ Accept if revised as suggested below
   _____ Do not accept for publication

2. Priority for publication:
   Low   High
   1   2   3   4   5

Areas you may wish to address in your review: (a) the manuscript's clarity of purpose; (b) the relevance, importance, and originality of the ideas presented; (c) the manuscript's organization; (d) the appropriateness of the topic; (e) the accuracy and timeliness of the content; (f) the interest the manuscript holds for the readers of RNJ. If the manuscript is a research study, address areas such as (a) the appropriateness of the methodology; (b) the adequacy of the literature review; (c) the significance of the findings' contribution to the field of practice.

Identify for the author(s) areas that should be expanded, condensed, or omitted. Suggest ways to strengthen the content or the style. Make specific comments that will help the author(s) revise the manuscript if necessary. Comments for the author(s):

Please sign your name: _____

Make any comments for the Editor *only* on the reverse side.

Return to Belinda Puetz, PhD RN, Editor, *Rehabilitation Nursing*, 11551 Dueling Oaks Court, Pensacola, FL 32514. Thank you.

---

*Reprinted with permission from the Association of Rehabilitation Nurses for Rehabilitation Nursing, 2506 Gross Point Road, Evanston, IL 60201.

INDEX